Nephrology Rounds

Nephrology Rounds

David J. Leehey, MD

Professor of Medicine
Loyola University of Chicago Medical Center
Maywood, Illinois
Associate Chief of Staff for Clinical Affairs
Veterans Administration Hospital
Hines, Illinois

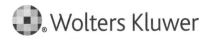. Wolters Kluwer

Philadelphia • Baltimore • New York • London
Buenos Aires • Hong Kong • Sydney • Tokyo

Acquisitions Editor: Kel McGowan
Product Development Editor: Leanne Vandetty
Marketing Manager: Stephanie Kindlick
Production Project Manager: Marian Bellus
Design Coordinator: Teresa Mallon
Manufacturing Coordinator: Beth Welsh
Prepress Vendor: S4Carlisle Publishing Services

9 8 7 6 5 4 3 2 1

Printed in China

Library of Congress Cataloging-in-Publication Data
Names: Leehey, David J., author.
Title: Nephrology rounds / David J. Leehey.
Description: First edition. | Philadelphia : Wolters Kluwer Health, [2016] |
  Includes bibliographical references and index.
Identifiers: LCCN 2015040255 | ISBN 9781496319708 (alk. paper)
Subjects: | MESH: Kidney Diseases—diagnosis—Case Reports. | Kidney
  Diseases—therapy—Case Reports. | Kidney Function Tests—Case Reports.
Classification: LCC RC903 | NLM WJ 302 | DDC 616.6/1—dc23 LC record available at http://
lccn.loc.gov/2015040255

RRS1512

To Patrick, Dorothy, and Roslyn Leehey

PREFACE

The learning of nephrology is challenging, and many medical students and resident physicians find nephrology to be a difficult subspecialty of medicine.

Over the course of teaching for more than three decades, I have noted that some areas of nephrology seem to be particularly difficult for trainees. In *Nephrology Rounds*, I have tried to focus on these areas, with particular attention to the principal concepts involved. Some examples include complex acid–base disturbances, sodium concentration disorders, and the utility of urine anion and osmolal gaps. I have also included some chapters where there is controversy about treatment, such as the use of bicarbonate to treat metabolic acidosis and phosphorus binders to treat hyperphosphatemia.

I would like to thank Dr. Todd Ing, Professor Emeritus of Nephrology at Loyola University Medical Center, Maywood, IL, who has been a mentor for my entire nephrology career, for reviewing and commenting upon the material in this book. I would also like to thank Drs. Mohamed Rahman, John Daugirdas, Ramin Sam, Julia Schneider, and Esho Georges, who gave valuable feedback on some of the book chapters.

Nephrology Rounds is meant to be a teaching and learning aid. It is not a comprehensive textbook. I hope that this modest book will facilitate the understanding of concepts that will stimulate the acquisition of knowledge and the application of knowledge.

David J. Leehey, MD

CONTENTS

Nephrology Rounds

How Is the Urinalysis Helpful in Patients with Kidney Disease?

In the past, urinalysis (UA) was a standard test done yearly in asymptomatic patients and routinely upon hospital admission. However, in the 1980s, this practice began to change owing to data indicating that routine UA on admission to the hospital rarely had an effect on patient care (Kroenke et al., 1986; Akin et al., 1987). The low yield of UA in unselected patients does not, however, contradict the statement that the UA is critically important in the diagnosis of renal and urologic disease. Indeed, it is generally the first test that the nephrologist looks at in evaluating acute kidney injury or chronic kidney disease. It would not be inaccurate to state that the UA is to Nephrology what the electrocardiogram (EKG) is to Cardiology (Sheets and Lyman, 1986).

There are three portions of a complete UA: the appearance of the urine, the dipstick evaluation, and the microscopic examination. A negative dipstick usually obviates the need for a microscopic examination. If dipstick proteinuria is detected, it should be quantitated by a random urine albumin-to-creatinine ratio (UACR) and/or urine protein-to-creatinine ratio (UPCR) (see Chapter 4).

In view of the importance of the UA in the clinical diagnosis of renal disease, it is surprising that many trainees and even some experienced physicians fail to appreciate the significance of its findings.

We will now take a tour through the UA.

APPEARANCE

The color of the urine should be assessed. Normal urine is clear (dilute) to yellow (concentrated). Macroscopic (gross) hematuria will make the urine appear red. Smoky red or cola-colored urine suggests hematuria of renal origin, typical of glomerulonephritis, but also seen with heme pigments in the absence of blood in the urine, as with myoglobinuria or hemoglobinuria. Dark yellow to orange urine is typical of bilirubinuria. Cloudy urine suggests pyuria or crystalluria (usually phosphates). Milky urine suggests chyluria (suggesting a lymphatic–urinary fistula). Some medications and foods will also change the color of urine (e.g., orange urine due to rifampin or phenazopyridine, blue/green urine due to methylene blue, light green urine after asparagus intake, light red urine after beet intake in susceptible persons).

DIPSTICK

- pH. The normal urine pH range is 4.5 to 8 (usually 5–7). A urine pH higher than 5.3 in the presence of metabolic acidosis raises the possibility of renal tubular acidosis (RTA). A very high urine pH (>8) suggests the presence of urea-splitting organisms (e.g., Proteus), in which cases production of ammonia (NH_3) will raise the urine pH.
- Specific gravity. The specific gravity is the weight of urine relative to distilled water and reflects the number and size (weight) of particles in urine. Osmolality is dependent on just the number of particles (solute concentration) in urine. Specific gravity is usually directly proportional to osmolality. However, iodinated contrast and, to a lesser extent, glucose and protein will increase specific gravity, but have little effect on osmolality. The normal range of urine specific gravity is 1.001 (very dilute) to 1.030 (very concentrated). Since the specific gravity of plasma is normally 1.010, a urine specific gravity of 1.010 indicates that the urine is neither concentrated nor dilute (isosthenuria). In an oliguric patient, a specific gravity of more than 1.020 suggests normal ability to concentrate urine and thus prerenal failure (decreased renal blood flow), whereas a specific gravity of about 1.010 suggests loss of tubular function (acute tubular necrosis/acute kidney injury). In a hyponatremic patient, an inappropriately high specific gravity (>1.010) suggests antidiuretic hormone (ADH) secretion, whereas in a hypernatremic patient, an inappropriately low specific gravity (<1.010) suggests diabetes insipidus (central or nephrogenic).
- Protein. The dipstick for protein detects primarily albumin. Normal urine usually has no protein by dipstick, but occasionally very concentrated urine will be trace or even 1+ positive for protein in healthy individuals. A positive dipstick should lead to a quantitative measurement. Classically, this was done by a 24-hour urine collection, but

since creatinine is excreted at a constant rate, the UACR or UPCR is sufficient in most patients (see Chapter 4). Simultaneous measurement of both UACR and UPCR is a good screening test for the presence of paraproteinuria, as in myeloma, in which case there will be a much more marked increase in urine total protein relative to urine albumin.

- Blood. A positive test indicates heme is present, which can be due to red blood cells (RBCs), myoglobinuria, or hemoglobinuria. Microscopic hematuria is hematuria in the absence of a visual change in color of the urine. As few as 2 to 3 RBCs/high-power field (hpf) may make the dipstick positive.
- Glucose. Normal urine does not contain glucose because of the reabsorption of filtered glucose by the proximal tubule. Glycosuria with elevated blood glucose indicates diabetes mellitus. Glycosuria with normal blood glucose indicates renal glycosuria, which may be isolated or associated with other evidence of proximal tubular dysfunction (phosphaturia, aminoaciduria, bicarbonaturia) (Fanconi syndrome).
- Ketones. Normally, there are no ketones in the urine. Ketonuria without ketoacidosis suggests starvation, low carbohydrate (such as Atkins) diet, or isopropyl alcohol ingestion. Ketonuria with ketoacidosis suggests diabetic or alcoholic ketoacidosis. Note that in some patients with ketoacidosis, the dipstick may be negative due to the reduction of acetoacetate to beta-hydroxybutyrate.
- Bilirubin. Normally, there is no bilirubin in the urine. If present, this suggests hepatobiliary disease (failure to conjugate and/or excrete bilirubin into the gut) or hemolysis (increased production of bilirubin from heme).
- Urobilinogen. Bilirubin is secreted in bile into the gut, where it is metabolized by microorganisms into urobilinogen. Urobilinogen is then absorbed and partially excreted into the urine. In the presence of liver disease, urobilinogen can accumulate in plasma and appear in the urine. Bilirubin without urobilinogen in the urine suggests biliary obstruction.
- Leukocyte esterase. This is an enzyme found in white blood cells (WBCs) and indicates the presence of pyuria, which can be due to either urinary tract infection (UTI) or inflammation (such as interstitial nephritis).
- Nitrite. Enterobacteria convert urinary nitrate to nitrite and therefore a positive test suggests UTI. Note that not all organisms make nitrite, so UTI may be present with a negative nitrite.

MICROSCOPIC EXAMINATION

- RBCs (Fig. 1.1). Hematuria requires evaluation if there are more than 3 RBCs/hpf on two out of three urinalyses, or more than 100 RBCs/hpf on one urine sample, or gross hematuria. In the absence of infection, if there is coexisting proteinuria, glomerulonephritis or renal vasculitis should be suspected.
- WBCs (Fig. 1.2). This is usually due to bacterial infection, but if sterile pyuria, one should exclude interstitial nephritis, nonbacterial infection, prostatitis, nephrolithiasis, and glomerulonephritis. Eosinophiluria suggests interstitial nephritis.

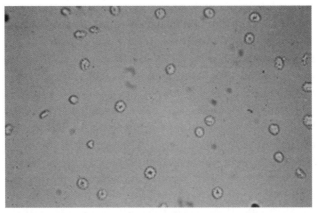

FIGURE 1.1 Red blood cells. (Image courtesy of Medcom, Inc. From Moinuddin IK, Leehey FJ. *Handbook of Nephrology*. Philadelphia, PA: Lippincott Williams & Wilkins; 2013.)

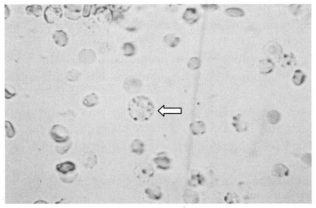

FIGURE 1.2 White blood cell (*arrow*). (Image courtesy of Medcom, Inc. From Moinuddin IK, Leehey FJ. *Handbook of Nephrology*. Philadelphia, PA: Lippincott Williams & Wilkins; 2013.)

- Squamous epithelial cells. Squamous epithelial cells from the skin surface or from the outer urethra or vagina in females can appear in urine, indicating possible contamination of the specimen with skin flora.
- Bacteria (Fig. 1.3). The presence of bacteria indicates possible infection depending on culture results.
- Yeast. These can indicate infection or colonization. The presence of pseudomycelia suggests infection. Risk factors include indwelling catheters, recent antibiotics, immunosuppression, and diabetes.
- Crystals. A number of different kinds of crystals can appear in the urine, including calcium oxalate dihydrate (envelopes) (Fig. 1.4), monohydrate (dumbbells), and calcium phosphate (amorphous—form in alkaline urine; in large amounts, may be associated with calcium phosphate kidney stones as may be seen in distal RTA). Uric acid crystals form in acid urine (pleomorphic, yellow/brown) (Fig. 1.5); when in large amounts, it suggests uric acid kidney stones or nephropathy. Cystine (hexagons) indicates cystinuria (Fig. 1.4). Magnesium ammonium phosphate (triple phosphate) ("coffin lids") can form struvite stones (a urea-splitting organism must be present to produce NH_3 and elevate urine pH) (Fig. 1.6).
- Casts. Urinary casts are formed in the distal nephron in the distal convoluted tubule (DCT) or collecting duct. Hyaline casts are composed primarily of a mucoprotein (Tamm–Horsfall protein) secreted by

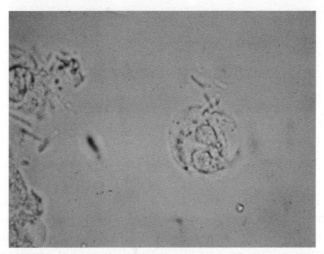

FIGURE 1.3 White blood cells and bacteria. (Image courtesy of Medcom, Inc. From Moinuddin IK, Leehey FJ. *Handbook of Nephrology*. Philadelphia, PA: Lippincott Williams & Wilkins; 2013.)

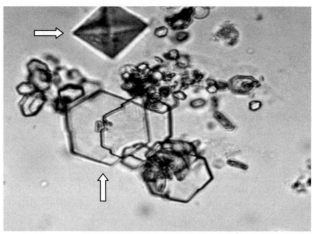

FIGURE 1.4 Calcium oxalate (*horizontal arrow*) and cystine (*vertical arrow*) crystals. (Image courtesy of Jessie Hano, MD. From Moinuddin IK, Leehey FJ. *Handbook of Nephrology.* Philadelphia, PA: Lippincott Williams & Wilkins; 2013.)

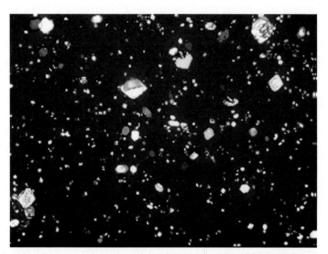

FIGURE 1.5 Uric acid crystals (polarized light). (Image courtesy of Subhash Popli, MD. From Moinuddin IK, Leehey FJ. *Handbook of Nephrology.* Philadelphia, PA: Lippincott Williams & Wilkins; 2013.)

tubule cells. They are formed in concentrated urine and can be seen in small numbers in healthy patients; large amounts suggest low urinary flow (prerenal or postrenal state) (Fig. 1.7). RBC casts are indicative of glomerulonephritis or vasculitis, with leakage of RBCs from glomeruli, or severe tubular damage (rare) (Fig. 1.8). WBC casts indicate acute

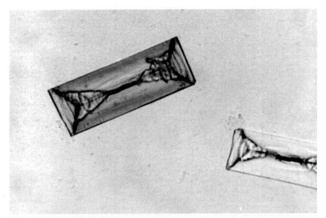

FIGURE 1.6 Triple phosphate crystals. (Image courtesy of Jessie Hano, MD. From Moinuddin IK, Leehey FJ. *Handbook of Nephrology*. Philadelphia, PA: Lippincott Williams & Wilkins; 2013.)

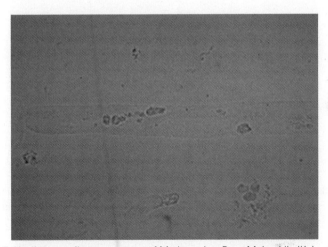

FIGURE 1.7 Hyaline cast. (Image courtesy of Medcom, Inc. From Moinuddin IK, Leehey FJ. *Handbook of Nephrology*. Philadelphia, PA: Lippincott Williams & Wilkins; 2013.)

pyelonephritis or kidney inflammation (usually tubulointerstitial) (Fig. 1.9). Granular casts are nonspecific, but indicate kidney disease (Fig. 1.10). Acute kidney injury (acute tubular necrosis) is characterized by pigmented granular ("muddy-brown") casts (Fig. 1.11). Renal tubular epithelial cell casts are seen in both acute and chronic kidney

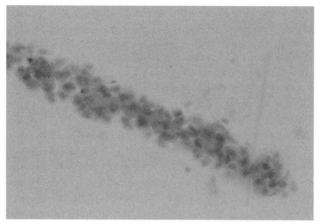

FIGURE 1.8 Red blood cell cast. (Image courtesy of T.S. Ing, MD. From Moinuddin IK, Leehey FJ. *Handbook of Nephrology.* Philadelphia, PA: Lippincott Williams & Wilkins; 2013.)

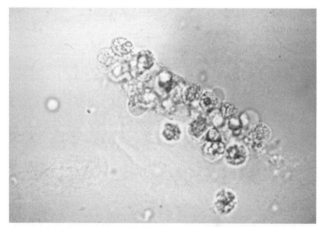

FIGURE 1.9 White blood cell cast. (Image courtesy of Jessie Hano, MD. From Moinuddin IK, Leehey FJ. *Handbook of Nephrology.* Philadelphia, PA: Lippincott Williams & Wilkins; 2013.)

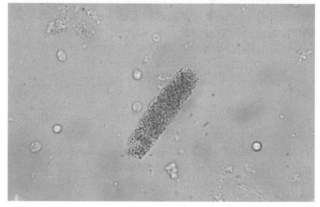

FIGURE 1.10 Granular cast. (Image courtesy of Medcom, Inc. From Moinuddin IK, Leehey FJ. *Handbook of Nephrology.* Philadelphia, PA: Lippincott Williams & Wilkins; 2013.)

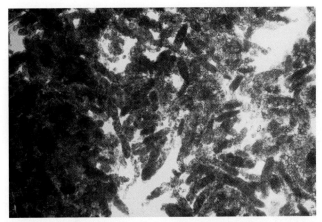

FIGURE 1.11 Muddy-brown casts. (Image by H. Richard Nesson, MD. From Dube GK, Brown RS. *Acute Tubular Necrosis*. Beth Israel Deaconess Medical Center; 2014, with permission.)

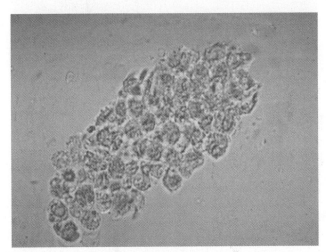

FIGURE 1.12 Renal tubular epithelial cell cast. (Image courtesy of Medcom, Inc. From Moinuddin IK, Leehey FJ. *Handbook of Nephrology*. Philadelphia, PA: Lippincott Williams & Wilkins; 2013.)

disease (Fig. 1.12). Broad waxy casts are seen in chronic kidney disease (Fig. 1.13). Fatty casts and oval fat bodies (lipid-laden macrophages) can be seen in nephrotic syndrome. Under polarizing light, characteristic "Maltese crosses" are seen (Fig. 1.14).

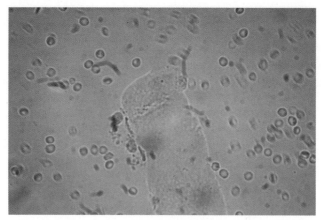

FIGURE 1.13 Broad waxy cast. (Image courtesy of Medcom, Inc. From Moinuddin IK, Leehey FJ. *Handbook of Nephrology.* Philadelphia, PA: Lippincott Williams & Wilkins; 2013.)

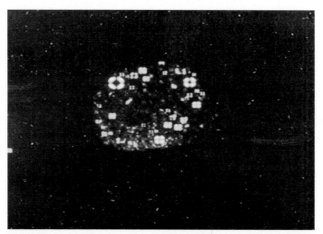

FIGURE 1.14 Oval fat body (polarized light). (Image courtesy of Jessie Hano, MD. From Moinuddin IK, Leehey FJ. *Handbook of Nephrology.* Philadelphia, PA: Lippincott Williams & Wilkins; 2013.)

CLINICAL SYNDROMES SUGGESTED BY THE URINALYSIS

See Table 1.1.

- A normal UA accompanied by an elevated serum creatinine suggests prerenal (decreased kidney blood flow) or postrenal failure (obstruction). Other less common conditions that can present like this are hypercalcemia, multiple myeloma (the dipstick will not detect paraproteins), hypertensive kidney disease (nephrosclerosis), and

Clinical Syndromes Suggested by the Urinalysis

Normal Urinalysis with Elevated Serum Creatinine	Hematuria/Proteinuria with or without Elevated Serum Creatinine ("Nephritis")	Massive Proteinuria with Bland Urine Sediment ("Nephrosis")
Prerenal failure	Exclude urinary tract	Diabetes
Postrenal failure	infection	Amyloid
Hypercalcemia	Glomerulonephritis:	Membranous nephropathy
Multiple myeloma	Lupus nephritis	Minimal change disease
Nephrosclerosis	IgA nephritis	Focal and segmental
Vasculopathies	Postinfectious	glomerulosclerosis
Ischemic nephropathy	glomerulonephritis	Less common entities
Calcineurin inhibitor toxicity	Peri-infectious (usually	include light-chain
	staphylococcal)	deposition disease,
	glomerulonephritis	immunotactoid
	Membranoproliferative	glomerulopathy, fibrillary
	glomerulonephritis	nephritis
	(MPGN) (usually	
	due to hepatitis	
	C with or without	
	cryoglobulinemia)	
	Rapidly progressive	
	glomerulonephritis	
	(RPGN) (including	
	antiglomerular	
	basement nephritis)	
	Vasculitis:	
	Granulomatous	
	polyangiitis	
	Other antineutrophil	
	cytoplasmic antibody	
	nephritides	
	Thrombotic	
	microangiopathy	

vasculopathies of medium-size vessels (polyarteritis nodosa, scleroderma, cholesterol emboli, ischemic nephropathy), although there is sometimes mild proteinuria.

- Hematuria/proteinuria with or without an elevated serum creatinine can be seen with UTI, in which case there will be pyuria and bacteriuria; in the absence of infection, this combination suggests glomerulonephritis or small-vessel vasculitis.
- Massive proteinuria with a bland urinary sediment (i.e., few cells, no cellular casts) suggests diabetes, amyloid, membranous nephropathy, minimal change disease, or focal and segmental glomerulosclerosis (FSGS).

PATIENT 1

A 70-year-old man with a long history of tobacco use presents to the ER with weakness. Examination reveals mild supine hypertension without orthostatic changes. There is an epigastric bruit. There is no edema. Laboratories reveal a serum creatinine of 5 mg/dL, which 1 month previously was 1 mg/dL. UA reveals the following:

Color yellow	Urobilinogen negative
pH 5.5	Leukocyte esterase negative
Specific gravity 1.025	Nitrite negative
Protein negative	WBC 2/hpf
Blood negative	RBC 3/hpf
Glucose negative	Bacteria negative
Ketones negative	Many hyaline casts
Bilirubin negative	Few granular casts

Q: What is the most likely diagnosis?

1. Acute glomerulonephritis
2. Acute interstitial nephritis
3. Acute tubular injury
4. Bilateral renal artery stenosis

A: The most likely diagnosis in this elderly male smoker with an epigastric bruit and acute azotemia is bilateral renal artery stenosis. Acute glomerulonephritis is excluded by the absence of proteinuria and hematuria, and interstitial nephritis is excluded by the absence of significant pyuria. Acute tubular injury would lead to isosthenuria, whereas this patient has concentrated urine. Bilateral renal artery stenosis leads to decreased renal blood flow and sodium and water retention by the kidneys. The patient ultimately underwent renal angiography, which revealed total occlusion of the right renal artery and 95% stenosis of the left renal artery. Angioplasty and stenting of the left renal artery resulted in improvement of renal function.

PATIENT 2

A 70-year-old woman with a history of hypertension and diabetes mellitus presents to the ER with weakness. Examination reveals normal vital signs but decreased skin turgor and evidence of malnutrition. There is no edema. Laboratories reveal a serum creatinine of 5 mg/dL, which 1 month previously was 1 mg/dL. Her complete blood count reveals pancytopenia and the serum calcium is elevated (11 mg/dL). UA reveals the following:

Color yellow	Urobilinogen negative
pH 5.5	Leukocyte esterase negative
Specific gravity 1.010	Nitrite negative
Protein negative	WBC 2/hpf
Blood negative	RBC 3/hpf
Glucose negative	Bacteria negative
Ketones negative	Many hyaline casts
Bilirubin negative	Few granular casts

Q: What is the most likely diagnosis?

1. Acute glomerulonephritis
2. Acute interstitial nephritis
3. Acute tubular injury
4. Multiple myeloma

A: The most likely diagnosis in this elderly female with pancytopenia, hypercalcemia, and acute azotemia is multiple myeloma. As in Patient 1, acute glomerulonephritis is excluded by the absence of proteinuria and hematuria, and interstitial nephritis is excluded by the absence of significant pyuria. Acute tubular injury is suggested by the finding of isosthenuria. However, this is not the most specific diagnosis that can be entertained. UACR was normal, but the UPCR was very elevated, suggesting the presence of a paraprotein in the urine. The diagnosis of myeloma was confirmed by serum and urine protein electrophoresis, serum-free light-chain assay, and bone marrow biopsy.

PATIENT 3

A 50-year-old man with a history of recent sore throat presents to the ER with leg swelling. Examination reveals severe hypertension (BP 190/120 mm Hg) and 2+ lower extremity edema. Laboratories reveal a serum creatinine of 5 mg/dL, which 1 month previously was 1 mg/dL. UA reveals the following:

Color cola-colored	Leukocyte esterase negative
pH 5.5	Nitrite negative
Specific gravity 1.020	WBC 2/hpf
Protein 3+	RBC 100/hpf
Blood 3+	Bacteria negative
Glucose negative	Few hyaline casts
Ketones negative	Many granular casts
Bilirubin negative	Occasional RBC casts
Urobilinogen negative	

Q: What is the most likely diagnosis?

1. Acute glomerulonephritis
2. Acute interstitial nephritis
3. Acute tubular injury
4. Multiple myeloma

A: The most likely diagnosis in this middle-aged man with hematuria with RBC casts and proteinuria, hypertension, acute azotemia, and a recent bout of pharyngitis is acute poststreptococcal glomerulonephritis (PSGN). In acute glomerulonephritis, the urine specific gravity (and urine osmolality) is usually elevated, suggesting a prerenal failure. This is because glomerular inflammation leads to decreased glomerular blood flow, resulting in decreased postglomerular perfusion and stimulation of sodium and water reabsorption by the kidneys. An antistreptolysin antibody (ASO) titer was positive. Renal biopsy confirmed the diagnosis.

PATIENT 4

A 50-year-old woman with a 20-year history of diabetes mellitus and a 5-year history of hypertension is seen in clinic. She complains of increasing leg swelling. Examination reveals moderate hypertension (BP 150/90 mm Hg) and 2+ lower extremity edema. Laboratories reveal a serum creatinine of 2 mg/dL, which 1 year previously was 1 mg/dL. UA reveals the following:

Color yellow	Urobilinogen negative
pH 5.5	Leukocyte esterase negative
Specific gravity 1.020	Nitrite negative
Protein 3+	WBC 2/hpf
Blood negative	RBC 3/hpf

Glucose negative   Bacteria negative
Ketones negative   Few hyaline casts
Bilirubin negative   No cellular casts

Q: What is the most likely diagnosis?

1. Acute glomerulonephritis
2. Acute interstitial nephritis
3. Acute tubular injury
4. Diabetic nephropathy

A: The most likely diagnosis in this middle-aged woman with a long history of diabetes and marked dipstick proteinuria but a bland urinary sediment (i.e., minimal cells, no cellular casts) is diabetic nephropathy (also called diabetic kidney disease). UPCR was markedly elevated (5,000 mg/g) and serum albumin was low (2.5 g/dL). Other causes of nephrotic syndrome can be considered, though the clinical picture is very consistent with diabetic kidney disease. Renal biopsy is not necessary in this patient.

References

Akin BV, Hubbell FA, Frye EB, et al. Efficacy of the routine admission urinalysis. *Am J Med.* 1987;82:719–722.

Kroenke K, Hanley JF, Copley JB, et al. The admission urinalysis: impact on patient care. *J Gen Intern Med.* 1986;1:238–242.

Sheets C, Lyman JL. Urinalysis. *Emerg Med Clin North Am.* 1986;4:263–280.

How Should Changes in Plasma Creatinine Be Interpreted?

2

Renal (glomerular) function is best determined by measuring the glomerular filtration rate (GFR). The most common methods utilize the endogenous substance creatinine, which is formed by the metabolism of creatine in skeletal muscle and excreted by glomerular filtration (although it is not a perfect marker of GFR, as there is also some tubular secretion). The plasma (or serum) creatinine concentration will reflect both the production rate of creatinine (which is proportional to muscle mass) and the excretion rate of creatinine (which depends on renal function). In the steady state, production will equal excretion, and plasma creatinine will be stable when repeatedly measured. Determination of GFR by creatinine clearance is discussed later in this chapter. Most of the time, clearance methods are not needed in clinical practice, and GFR is estimated from the plasma creatinine concentration using various formulae, as will also be discussed later in this chapter.

CHRONIC RENAL FAILURE (CHRONIC KIDNEY DISEASE)

By definition, a patient with chronic kidney disease (CKD) has had kidney disease for months to years (at least 3 months by standard definitions) (Table 2.1). GFR may or may not be impaired. By current convention, if estimated GFR (eGFR) is moderately impaired (30–59 mL/min/1.73 m^2), this is termed *stage 3 CKD*, whereas more severe impairment (15–29 mL/min/1.73 m^2) and very severe impairment (<15 mL/min/1.73 m^2) are termed *stage 4 CKD* and *stage 5 CKD*, respectively. As GFR decreases, plasma creatinine will progressively rise, generally over months to years. The change in plasma creatinine is very slow, and thus the concentration

TABLE 2.1	Chronic Kidney Disease versus Acute Kidney Disease

Chronic Kidney Disease	Acute Kidney Disease
Duration months to years (>3 mo)	Duration hours to days
Nonoliguric	Nonoliguric or oliguric
GFR usually impaired but can be normal	GFR always impaired, usually severely
Progressive linear decline in GFR over months to years is typical (though it can be slowed by treatment)	Linear increase in plasma creatinine (severity can be assessed by "delta creatinine")
Exponential increase in plasma creatinine as renal function declines	Low urine-to-plasma (U/P) creatinine ratio (in an oliguric patient, the lower the U/P creatinine ratio, the more severe the disease)
Can use eGFR formulae to estimate GFR	Cannot use eGFR formulae to estimate GFR

will be stable if measured daily. (If it rises every day, this is *acute* or *acute-on-chronic* renal failure.) This is because, in CKD with diminished GFR, production still equals excretion of creatinine, though at an increased plasma creatinine level. As CKD progresses, there will be an exponential increase in plasma creatinine as renal function declines. This is shown in Figure 2.1. The reason for the exponential increase merits further discussion.

Determination of GFR in CKD by Creatinine-Based Methods
Measured Creatinine Clearance
When a substance is cleared from the blood by glomerular filtration, the excretion rate of the substance (assuming no secretion or reabsorption by the tubules) will equal the volume of plasma that is totally cleared of the substance. Therefore,

$$\text{Plasma concentration} \times \text{Clearance} = \text{Urine concentration} \times \text{Urinary flow rate, or}$$

$$\text{Clearance} = (\text{Urine concentration} \times \text{Urinary flow rate})/ \text{Plasma concentration} [(UV/P)]$$

For example, if a patient excretes 1,440 mg of creatinine in 24 hours (1 mg/min) and the plasma concentration is 1 mg/dL (0.01 mg/mL), the creatinine clearance = 1 mg/min/0.01 mg/mL = 100 mL/min.

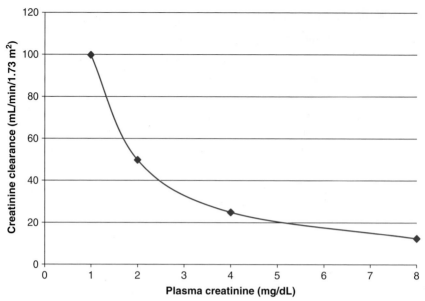

FIGURE 2.1 Inverse relationship between plasma creatinine and creatinine clearance in CKD.

Creatinine-Based Formulae

(*Note:* All of these formulae require a steady-state [stable] level of plasma creatinine, and cannot be used in patients whose renal function is rapidly changing.)

Inverse Creatinine. Since creatinine clearance (CCr) is inversely proportional to plasma creatinine (PCr), that is, CCr ~ 1/PCr, a rough approximation of renal function can be obtained in this manner. For example, if CCr is 100 mL/min when PCr is 1 mg/dL, then CCr would be 50 mL/min when PCr is 2 mg/dL, and 25 mL/min when PCr is 4 mg/dL. Therefore, there is an exponential relationship between creatinine clearance (an estimate of GFR) and plasma creatinine (Fig. 2.1).

Cockroft–Gault Equation. This formula was developed empirically during the 1970s by Cockroft and Gault (1976):

$$\text{Creatinine clearance (mL/min)} = [(140 - \text{Age}) \times \text{Body weight (kg)}/ 72 \times \text{Plasma creatinine}] \times 0.85$$
$$\text{(if female)}$$

Other modifications of this formula have been made (e.g., using correction factors of 0.8 for paraplegia and 0.6 for quadriplegia). It has now essentially been replaced by formulae for eGFR in laboratory medicine, although it still has value as it is easy to calculate at the bedside and can be useful for estimating GFR in special populations (e.g., spinal cord–injured patients).

MDRD Formulae. These formulae were developed from data obtained in the Modification of Diet in Renal Disease (MDRD) Study (Levey et al., 1989). As this study did not include many non-Caucasian or diabetic patients and was based on subjects with fairly advanced renal failure, the CKD-EPI (Chronic Kidney Disease Epidemiology Collaboration) equation was subsequently developed on the basis of data from several clinical trials including a much broader range of patients, and is more applicable to patients with normal or near-normal renal function (Levey et al., 2009).

MDRD formula: eGFR (mL/min/1.73 m^2)
$$= 186 \times \text{SCr}^{-1.154} \times \text{Age}^{-0.203} \times 0.742 \text{ (if female)} \times 1.21 \text{ (if black)}$$

CKD-EPI formula: eGFR (mL/min/1.73 m^2)
$$= 141 \times \min(\text{SCr}/k,1)^{\alpha} \times \max(\text{SCr}/k,1)^{-1.209}$$
$$\times 0.993^{\text{Age}} \times 1.018 \text{ (if female)} \times 1.159 \text{ (if black)}$$

where SCr is serum creatinine (mg/dL), k is 0.7 for females and 0.9 for males, α is -0.329 for females and -0.411 for males, min indicates the minimum of SCr/k or 1, and max indicates the maximum of SCr/k or 1.

The MDRD and CKD-EPI formulae are available as Web-based and downloadable calculators at various websites, including www.hdcn.com, www.nephron.com, and www.qxmd.com. Note that these formulae utilize serum creatinine (SCr), although this can be substituted by plasma creatinine (PCr). A coupled enzymatic assay that meets the isotope dilution mass spectrometry (IDMS) standard should be used to measure creatinine.

In all of these formulae, the plasma creatinine is in the denominator, just as it is in the classic clearance formula (UV/P), showing the inverse relationship between plasma creatinine and GFR.

ACUTE RENAL FAILURE (ACUTE KIDNEY DISEASE)

Acute renal failure is defined as a rapid decline in kidney function over a period of hours to days (as opposed to CKD, where kidney function worsens over months to years) (Table 2.1). Acute worsening of kidney function will lead to a rapid increase in plasma creatinine concentration. The reason for the worsening of kidney function must be deduced by the clinician. However, the rate of change of plasma creatinine is helpful in clinical practice in assessing the severity of acute renal failure. If kidney function abruptly ceases or declines to very low levels, plasma creatinine will generally increase at a rate of 1 to 1.5 mg/dL/day. This daily change in plasma creatinine is sometimes called "delta creatinine" on rounds. With severe acute renal failure, there will be a linear increase in plasma creatinine concentration due to continued production of creatinine in the face of minimal excretion. If kidney function begins to improve, the "delta creatinine" will slow and then eventually approach zero (at which point, production again equals excretion); continued improvement in kidney function will lead to excretion in excess of production and a fall in plasma creatinine concentration (a negative "delta creatinine"). Figure 2.2 demonstrates this in pictorial form.

Monitoring changes in "delta creatinine" is very helpful in assessing the severity of acute renal failure and the likelihood of requiring dialysis. Creatinine clearance is not typically used in the setting of acute renal failure because of difficulties in determining clearance in the face of low urine output. However, the urine-to-plasma creatinine ratio on a random urine specimen is easily obtained and can be very useful. As an example,

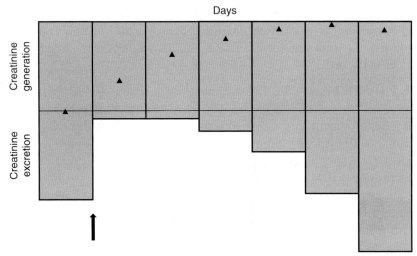

FIGURE 2.2 *Triangles* depict plasma creatinine levels. The *arrow* indicates the timing of renal insult (in this case, contrast exposure). Over the next 2 days, creatinine excretion is markedly impaired, and plasma creatinine rises in a linear fashion (the absolute daily increment depends on the creatinine generation rate). On day 3, renal function begins to improve (increase in creatinine excretion), and the rate of rise of plasma creatinine begins to decrease. However, plasma creatinine does not peak until day 5, at which time creatinine excretion again equals creatinine generation. Plasma creatinine begins to decline only when creatinine excretion exceeds creatinine generation.

if the urine creatinine is 30 mg/dL and the patient is oliguric, excreting only 400 mL of urine daily, the creatinine excretion would be only 120 mg/day, far less than the production rate (usually about 15 mg/kg/day in women and 20 mg/kg/day in men, although it is quite variable depending on muscle mass). In this case, one would predict that the plasma creatinine will rise rapidly. On the other hand, if the urine creatinine is 300 mg/dL, and the patient is again excreting 400 mL of urine daily, this translates to a daily excretion of 1,200 mg of creatinine, which will be approximately the same as the daily production, and plasma creatinine may rise little if at all. The former situation is typical of acute kidney injury (AKI), formerly termed acute tubular necrosis (ATN), whereas the latter is typical of prerenal conditions such as volume depletion, cardiorenal syndrome, and hepatorenal syndrome (in the absence of superimposed kidney injury).

PATIENT 1

A 22-year-old medical student is taking renal physiology, and as part of the course, he submits a plasma sample and a 24-hour urine sample for determination of creatinine clearance. His plasma creatinine is 1 mg/dL, and his 24-hour urine sample contains 1,440 mg of creatinine in a volume of 1 L.

Q1: What is his creatinine clearance?

A1: His creatinine clearance (CCr) can be determined by the following formula:

$$\text{Clearance} = (\text{Urine concentration} \times \text{Urinary flow rate})/\text{Plasma concentration } [(\text{UV}/\text{P})]$$

$$\text{CCr} = (1{,}440 \text{ mg/L} \times 1 \text{ L}/1{,}440 \text{ min})/1 \text{ mg/dL} = 1 \text{ mg/min}/0.01 \text{ mg/mL} = 100 \text{ mL/min}$$

Q2: Ten years later, he is a nephrology attending, and decides to recheck his plasma creatinine. He is dismayed to find that it is now 2 mg/dL. He repeats the test several times over the next several days and gets the same result each time. What is his 24-hour urine creatinine now?

A2: The correct answer is that it is the same as it was 10 years earlier, providing he did not lose or gain muscle mass in the interim. Since plasma creatinine is stable, he is in a steady state and thus excreting all of the creatinine produced. It can be seen that his CCr will now be 50 mL/min.

PATIENT 2

A 65-year-old man undergoes coronary artery bypass graft (CABG) surgery, after which he develops AKI. His plasma creatinine was 1 mg/dL preoperatively. On the first postoperative day, his plasma creatinine is 2 mg/dL. On the second postoperative day, it is 2.8 mg/dL, and on the third postoperative day, it is 3.2 mg/dL. He is nonoliguric and not fluid overloaded, and has no electrolyte abnormalities.

Q1: Is his renal function worsening or improving on postoperative day 3?

A1: Even though his plasma creatinine is continuing to increase, the "delta creatinine" is decreasing (day 1: 1 mg/dL; day 2: 0.8 mg/dL; day 3: 0.4 mg/dL). Therefore, his renal function is improving.

Q2: Do you predict that he will need dialysis?

A2: No. His renal function is expected to continue to improve, providing there are no additional renal insults. His plasma creatinine will probably peak at about 3.5 mg/dL and then begin to decline.

References

Cockroft DW, Gault MH. Prediction of creatinine clearance from plasma creatinine. *Nephron.* 1976;16:31–41.

Levey AS, Berg RL, Gassman JJ, et al. Creatinine filtration, secretion, and excretion during progressive renal disease. *Kidney Int.* 1989;36(suppl 27):S73–S80.

Levey AS, Stevens LA, Schmid CH, et al.; CKD-EPI (Chronic Kidney Disease Epidemiology Collaboration). A new equation to estimate glomerular filtration rate. *Ann Intern Med.* 2009;150(9): 604–612.

3

What Is Fractional Excretion and How Does Measuring It Help in Clinical Practice?

DERIVATION OF THE FORMULA

Fractional excretion is a term that nephrologists frequently use in clinical practice (Schrier, 1988a, b). What exactly does it mean? Forgetting the formulae for now, fractional excretion of a substance is the amount of that substance that is excreted into the urine relative to the amount of that substance that is filtered by the kidney.

$$\text{Fractional excretion} = \text{Amount excreted/Amount filtered}$$

Since fractional excretion is generally expressed as a percentage and not a fraction, it can be defined simply as the percentage of the filtered substance that is excreted into the urine.

Now we will derive the formula. For example, take fractional excretion of sodium (FENa). The amount of sodium excreted is the product of the urine sodium concentration and the urine flow rate, that is, $UNa \times V$. Since sodium is freely filterable, the amount of sodium filtered is the product of the plasma sodium concentration and the glomerular filtration rate (GFR), that is, $PNa \times GFR$. Therefore,

$$FENa = (UNa \times V)/(PNa \times GFR)$$

Substituting creatinine clearance ($UCr \times V/PCr$) for GFR (a pretty good approximation) results in as follows:

$$FENa = (UNa \times V)/[PNa \times (UCr \times V/PCr)]$$

The *V* terms cancel out, resulting in the following equation:

$$\text{FENa} = \text{UNa}/(\text{PNa} \times \text{UCr}/\text{PCr})$$

Multiplying both numerator and denominator by PCr/UCr results in the most commonly used formula:

$$\text{FENa} = (\text{UNa}/\text{PNa}) \times (\text{PCr}/\text{UCr}) \times 100$$

Do not forget to multiply by 100, to convert from a fraction to a percentage!

WHAT IS THE FRACTIONAL EXCRETION OF SODIUM IN HEALTHY PEOPLE?

Most healthy people on standard American diets have a FENa of approximately equal to 1%. Let us see why.

A typical American diet contains about 6 g of sodium daily. How many millimoles (mmol) or milliequivalents (mEq) is 6 g? First of all, since sodium is univalent (has a single charge, in this case, positive), millimoles = milliequivalents. For the remainder of this discussion, we are going to use millimoles, since milliequivalents cannot be used for nonionic (uncharged) analytes. However, in other chapters, we will use milliequivalents sometimes and millimoles at other times for ion concentrations.

The molecular weight of sodium is 23. Therefore, 1 mmol = 23 mg. (Remember this mantra: A millimole is the molecular weight in milligrams.)

Thus, 6 g or 6,000 mg sodium = 6,000 mg/(23 mg/mmol) = 261 mmol

In the steady state, what is ingested must be excreted. Most of the excretion will be in the urine. For the sake of simplicity, let us assume other losses (stool, sweat) are minimal and that 250 mmol/day of sodium appears in the urine, and that there is 2 L/day of urine excretion. The urine sodium concentration is thus 125 mmol/L.

Remember that daily urine sodium excretion (in this case, 250 mmol) is urine concentration (125 mmol/L) × urine flow rate (2 L/day), and thus the numerator of the FENa formula. Now, how about the denominator of the formula? The normal creatinine clearance is about 180 L/day (125 mL/min). This means that 180 L of plasma is completely cleared of creatinine by the kidneys in 1 day. The normal plasma sodium concentration is 140 mmol/L. Therefore, the amount of sodium filtered equals 180 L/day × 140 mmol/L = 25,200 mmol/day.

$$\text{FENa} = (250 \text{ mmol}/25{,}200 \text{ mmol}) \times 100 \approx 1\%$$

FRACTIONAL EXCRETION OF SODIUM IN PATHOPHYSIOLOGIC STATES

Chronic Kidney Disease

Many patients with chronic kidney disease (CKD) are unaware of their condition and are referred to a nephrologist when the GFR is found to be low in the absence of specific symptoms and signs.

PATIENT 1

A 50-year-old man with moderately severe CKD (estimated GFR by creatinine-based formula of 25 mL/min/1.73 m^2) is seen in clinic. His physical examination is normal and he has no peripheral edema.

Q: What is the expected FENa?

A: As stated earlier, the typical American diet contains about 6 g of sodium per day. If a patient with CKD continues to ingest a typical diet (a good assumption for many patients!) and has not developed progressive edema, this means that the daily amount of sodium excreted still approximates the daily dietary intake of sodium. Sodium excreted thus has not changed; however, the amount of filtered sodium must decrease proportional to the GFR. In this instance, if the GFR is 25% of normal, that is, 45 L/day rather than 180 L/day, the amount of sodium filtered will be 45 L/day $\times$ 140 mmol/L = 6,300 mmol/day.

$$FENa = (250 \text{ mmol}/63{,}000 \text{ mmol}) \times 100 \approx 4\%$$

One can see that, assuming no change in dietary sodium intake, the FENa will double for every halving of GFR. With very severe CKD (e.g., GFR 10% of normal), FENa may be as high as 10%. Of course, hopefully such a patient has learned to restrict his or her sodium intake so that it will not actually be that high. Diseased kidneys usually have an impaired ability to excrete ingested sodium, so the development of sodium overload is common as the GFR declines unless the patient restricts sodium intake.

Congestive Heart Failure

Most patients with congestive heart failure (CHF) do learn to restrict sodium in their diet (otherwise they end up in the hospital with decompensated heart failure).

PATIENT 2

A 50-year-old man with severe CHF (ejection fraction, 20%) is seen in clinic. He has normal renal function. His body weight is stable and he has chronic mild peripheral edema. He states that he is following a 2-g sodium (no added salt) diet.

Q1: What is the expected FENa?

A1: Although this patient has edema, his stable body weight indicates that he has a stable extracellular fluid volume, so the daily amount of sodium excreted will again approximate the daily dietary intake of sodium. In this case, daily urine sodium excretion will be 2,000 mg/ (23 mg/mmol) = 87 mmol. Therefore,

$$FENa = (87 \text{ mmol}/25,200 \text{ mmol}) \times 100 \approx 0.33\%$$

Because of his peripheral edema, he is prescribed a loop diuretic (furosemide 20 mg twice daily). When he returns to clinic in 2 weeks, he states that he has lost 10 lb (about 4 kg) since the last visit. Most of this weight loss occurred in the first week after starting the furosemide, and his weight has been stable for the past several days. His edema has resolved. He has been taking the diuretic regularly, but did not take it the morning of the clinic visit.

Q2: What will the FENa be at the time of the clinic visit?

A2: Administration of an effective dose of diuretic will lead to increased excretion of salt and water. Indeed, if the patient took the furosemide on the morning of the follow-up visit, FENa would be expected to be higher than before (probably >1%). However, since he did not take it, the FENa would probably still be approximately equal to 0.33% or even less. Why? The common brand name for furosemide is Lasix, the brand name meaning "lasts 6 hours." The effect of the last dose of Lasix taken the previous day has dissipated by the following morning. Now antinatriuretic forces due to diuretic-induced volume depletion in conjunction with CHF are strongly signaling the kidney to reabsorb sodium.

Patients (and many doctors as well) get confused by diuretics. It is very common for patients to say that they cannot take diuretics because it makes them urinate too much! It is true that short-acting loop diuretics such as Lasix have a rapid onset of action and will have a noticeable effect on urine volume, because the loop of Henle normally reabsorbs as much as 20% of the filtered salt and water load. However, continued loss of salt and water into the urine in excess of intake over a period of weeks is decidedly unusual. This is because the remaining nephron segments will increase their sodium and water reabsorption to "brake" the losses caused by blockade of loop transport. The mechanisms of such diuretic adaptation are complex, but the important thing to realize from a clinical standpoint is that if this did not occur diuretics would lead to progressive volume depletion and hypovolemic shock! Occasionally, excess salt and water losses resulting in clinically significant volume depletion can occur, particularly in one of the following scenarios:

1. Continued diuretic intake in the presence of a sudden decrease in salt and water intake or increased extrarenal losses of salt and water, such as with vomiting or diarrhea; or
2. If two different types of diuretics (e.g., a loop and distal tubule diuretic) are used simultaneously.

A more frequent problem is failure to take the diuretic regularly, which leads to "diuretic rebound" and worsening of edema (Chan et al., 1979). This occurs because now the adaptive increase in sodium and water reabsorption is no longer opposed by the diuretic effect.

FRACTIONAL EXCRETION OF OTHER SUBSTANCES

Although fractional excretion of sodium is the most common fractional excretion used in clinical practice, one can measure the fractional excretion of any substance that is freely filtered by the glomerulus.

For instance, let us consider fractional excretion of potassium (FEK). As with dietary sodium intake, dietary potassium intake varies substantially among individuals. A daily intake of about 4 g is typical. The molecular weight of potassium is 39. Therefore, 1 mmol = 39 mg.

Thus, 4 g or 4,000 mg potassium = 4,000 mg/39 mg/mmol = 103 mmol

Again, for the sake of simplicity, let us assume other losses (stool, sweat) are minimal and that 100 mmol/day of potassium appears in the urine, and that there is 2 L/day of urine excretion. The urine potassium concentration in this case would be 50 mmol/L.

Remember that daily urine potassium excretion (in this case, 100 mmol) is urine concentration (50 mmol/L) $\times$ urine flow rate (2 L/day), and thus the numerator of the FEK formula. The denominator of the formula will be the amount of potassium filtered, which equals 180 L/day $\times$ 4 mmol/L = 720 mmol/day.

$$FEK = (50 \text{ mmol}/720 \text{ mmol}) \times 100 \approx 7\%$$

Similar calculations can be made to determine fractional excretion of chloride, bicarbonate, urea, calcium, phosphorus, magnesium, uric acid, and even endogenous lithium. (The latter is a good marker of proximal tubular function, since lithium is reabsorbed solely by the proximal tubule; however, this measurement is not widely available.) Fractional excretion of urea is commonly measured to assess tubular function in patients taking diuretics (which interfere with tubular sodium but not urea transport) (Carvounis et al., 2002). One caveat is that in order to measure fractional excretion of magnesium (FEMg), one must estimate plasma ionized magnesium by multiplying plasma magnesium by 0.7. (70% of plasma magnesium is in the ionized form and 30% is bound to proteins, predominantly albumin.) Similarly, to measure fractional excretion of calcium (FECa), one cannot use plasma total calcium, since this measurement includes both filterable calcium and calcium bound to proteins and thus unable to be filtered by the glomeruli. Normally about 60% of total calcium is freely filterable (50% ionized and 10% complexed to plasma anions).

Expected fractional excretions of various substances in various clinical conditions are shown in Tables 3.1 and 3.2.

TABLE 3.1 Expected Fractional Excretions of Sodium (FENa), Chloride (FECl), and Urea Nitrogen (FEUN)

	FENa/FECl		FEUN	
	Low (<1%)	High (>1%)	Low (<35%)	High (>35%)
Volume depletion (extrarenal loss)	+		+	
Volume depletion (renal loss)		+	+	
Effective volume depletion (CHF, cirrhosis)	+		+	
Chronic kidney disease		+		+
Diuretics (during drug administration)		+	+	
Diuretics (after drug cessation)	+		+	

TABLE 3.2	Expected Fractional Excretions of Potassium (FEK) and Magnesium (FEMg)			
	FEK		**FEMg**	
	Low (<10%)	High (>10%)	Low (<2%)	High (>2%)
Mineral depletion (extrarenal loss)	+		+	
Mineral depletion (renal loss)		+		+

References

Carvounis CP, Nisar S, Guro-Razuman S. Significance of the fractional excretion of urea in the differential diagnosis of acute renal failure. *Kidney Int.* 2002;62:2223–2229.

Chan MK, Sweny P, Varghese Z, et al. Diuretic escape and rebound oedema in renal allograft recipients. *Br Med J.* 1979;1(6178):1604–1605.

Schrier RW. Pathogenesis of sodium and water retention in high-output and low-output cardiac failure, nephrotic syndrome, cirrhosis, and pregnancy (1). *N Engl J Med.* 1988a;319:1065–1072.

Schrier RW. Pathogenesis of sodium and water retention in high-output and low-output cardiac failure, nephrotic syndrome, cirrhosis, and pregnancy (2). *N Engl J Med.* 1988b;319:1127–1134.

4

What Is Urine Albumin-to-Creatinine Ratio? (Or Is It Protein-to-Creatinine Ratio?)

The amount of urinary albumin or protein is an important diagnostic and prognostic factor in patients with kidney disease (Peterson et al., 1995; Bigazzi et al., 1998; Leehey et al., 2005). Many trainees are uncertain about how to interpret the urine albumin-to-creatinine ratio (UACR) or urine protein-to-creatinine ratio (UPCR). Possibly, some of this confusion can be blamed on the nephrology community, as literature and guidelines sometimes incorporate one measurement, sometimes the other, and sometimes both. Laboratories also vary in their testing practices, with some not measuring UACR if there is overt (i.e., dipstick-positive) proteinuria. This practice stems from the fact that in the past urinary albumin measurement was generally done by immunoassay, which was more laborious and expensive than urinary total protein measurement. With current autoanalyzers, however, it is usually very simple and inexpensive to run and report both UACR and UPCR on the same specimen. We generally use both UACR and UPCR in the initial evaluation of the patient with proteinuria. In those with established proteinuric kidney disease, we typically follow just the UPCR.

First, let us review some concepts. Most proteins, that is, albumin and globulins, are too big to pass through the normal glomerular filtration barrier in substantial amounts, and thus persistent proteinuria is usually a sign that the glomeruli are damaged. Glomerular proteinuria can be transient if it results from increased hydrostatic pressure (such as in congestive heart failure) or variables such as exercise or fever. It is pathologic only if the proteinuria is persistent. There are other smaller molecular weight proteins in the plasma that are filtered and normally reabsorbed by the renal tubules, including light chains (polyclonal), alpha-1-microglobulin, and beta-2-microglobulin. Impaired tubular reabsorption of these filtered proteins indicates tubular damage ("tubular proteinuria"). Finally, "overflow proteinuria" occurs in situations in which abnormally large concentrations of small proteins (such as monoclonal light chains, hemoglobin, or myoglobin) are produced and are freely filtered by the glomerulus, overwhelming the capacity of the renal tubules to completely reabsorb and catabolize these proteins, so they appear in the urine. Typically, overflow proteinuria is due to the overproduction of monoclonal proteins, sometimes called "paraproteins."

URINE ALBUMIN-TO-CREATININE RATIO AND PROTEIN-TO-CREATININE RATIO

Since albumin, protein, and creatinine are usually excreted at a constant rate, measurement of ratios in a random urine specimen can generally be substituted for 24-hour urine measurements. Assuming renal function is stable (i.e., steady state), the rate of urinary creatinine excretion reflects the generation rate of creatinine by muscle. It can vary greatly depending on muscle mass (0.3–3 g/day, with a median of about 1 g/day). If excretion of 1 g/day is assumed, then a UACR or UPCR of 1 g/g would indicate 1 g of daily albumin or protein excretion. Note that some labs measure UACR and UPCR as milligrams per gram, so this ratio would then be 1,000 mg/g.

UACR was introduced into clinical medicine to assess low amounts of albumin excretion that cannot be detected by standard urine dipsticks for protein (so-called *microalbumin*). (The term *microalbumin* has also led to some confusion and is now being replaced by the more appropriate term *albumin*.) The upper limit of urinary albumin excretion is 30 mg/day. Excretion of between 30 and 300 mg of albumin in the urine per day is commonly observed in a number of clinical conditions, including uncontrolled diabetes and hypertension, and does not necessarily imply kidney disease. Overt albuminuria is the excretion of more than 300 mg of albumin in the urine per day (this amount is detectable by dipstick, i.e., "dipstick proteinuria"). If persistent, it indicates the presence of glomerular disease.

Healthy people excrete some proteins in their urine. It is generally accepted that about 20% of these urinary proteins are albumin, with the remainder globulins, including Tamm–Horsfall proteins. In most laboratories, the upper limits for albumin and protein excretion are 30 and

TABLE 4.1	Chronic Kidney Disease Stages Based on eGFR and Albumin Excretion Rate (AER)	
GFR Stage	**eGFR (mL/min/1.73 m^2)**	**Description**
G1	>90	Normal
G2	60–89	Slightly decreased
G3a	45–59	Mild to moderately decreased
G3b	30–44	Moderately to severely decreased
G4	15–29	Severely decreased
G5	<15	Kidney failure (G5d, on dialysis, or end-stage renal disease)
Albuminuria Stage	**AER (mg/day)**	**Description**
A1	<30	Normal to slightly increased
A2	30–300	Moderately increased
A3	>300	Severely increased ("overt albuminuria")

150 mg/day, respectively, although, depending on the method, up to 300 mg/day of protein excretion may be normal in healthy people (Leischner et al., 2006). Although arbitrary, usual cutoffs for "overt albuminuria" and "overt proteinuria" are 300 mg/day (or 300 mg/g creatinine) and 500 mg/day (or 500 mg/g creatinine), respectively.

A disproportionately elevated UPCR versus UACR suggests either tubular proteinuria or overflow proteinuria. For instance, if the UACR is 15 mg/g but the UPCR is 500 mg/g, tubular or overflow proteinuria should be suspected, and should raise the suspicion for paraproteinuria.

The UACR has prognostic value in patients with chronic kidney disease (CKD). In general, the higher the UACR, the worse the prognosis, that is, the greater the likelihood and rate of renal progression. For this reason, staging of CKD now takes into account both estimated glomerular filtration rate (eGFR) and UACR (Table 4.1).

PATIENT 1

A 65-year-old man is referred to the renal clinic for evaluation of proteinuria and edema. Review of the record reveals that there is a positive (2–3+) dipstick for protein on multiple urinalyses (UAs). The urine microalbumin is 1,500 mg/L.

Q1: What kind of proteinuria does this patient have and how severe is the proteinuria?

A1: This patient has albuminuria based on both the UA and the concentration of albumin in the urine. This suggests that the patient has glomerular proteinuria.

Q2: How much albumin is the patient excreting in the urine?

A2: Unfortunately, we cannot really assess that without knowing the patient's urine volume. The concentration of albumin in the urine (assessed by either dipstick or urine albumin concentration) reflects both the albumin excretion rate and the concentration of the urine. To correct for urine concentration, typically urine creatinine concentration is employed. The correct thing to do in this patient is to order a UACR and UPCR. This test reveals the UACR to be 4,500 mg/g creatinine and the UPCR to be 5,000 mg/g creatinine.

Q3: Was there any reason to measure both UACR and UPCR in this patient?

A3: The answer is a qualified yes. Just because there is albuminuria does not exclude the presence of globulins and even paraproteins in the urine. In this case, the fact that UPCR is only slightly greater than the UACR suggests that most (~90%) of the urinary proteins are albumin and that we are dealing with glomerular and not tubular or overflow proteinuria.

   Why not just do a urine protein electrophoresis on every patient with proteinuria to make sure they do not have paraproteinuria? True, this is a more definitive test, but adds expense and probably has no added value in the aforementioned situation.

PATIENT 2

A 70-year-old female with anemia, hypercalcemia, and a recent left hip fracture was admitted for worsening renal function accompanied by rib and back pain. The UA shows 1+ protein but is otherwise unremarkable. The UACR is 60 mg/g and the UPCR is 2,000 mg/g.

   In this case, there is a marked discrepancy between the UACR and UPCR, with UPCR >> UACR. This should always suggest a paraproteinuria. The urinary protein electrophoresis (UPEP) and immunofixation showed the presence of a monoclonal IgG kappa spike and a large amount of kappa light chains. There was also a monoclonal IgG kappa spike and a moderate amount of free kappa light chains in the plasma. Bone marrow biopsy confirmed the diagnosis of multiple myeloma.

References

Bigazzi R, Bianchi S, Baldari D, et al. Microalbuminuria predicts cardiovascular events and renal insufficiency in patients with essential hypertension. *J Hypertens*. 1998;16:1325–1333.

Leehey DJ, Kramer HJ, Daoud TM, et al. Progression of kidney disease in type 2 diabetes: beyond blood pressure control—an observational study. *BMC Nephrol*. 2005;6:8.

Leischner MP, Naratadam GO, Hou SH, et al. Evaluation of proteinuria in healthy live kidney donor candidates. *Transplant Proc*. 2006;38(9):2796–2797.

Peterson JC, Adler S, Burkart JM, et al. Blood pressure control, proteinuria, and the progression of renal disease. The modification of diet in renal disease study. *Ann Intern Med*. 1995;123:754–762.

5

What Is the Meaning of the Urine-to-Plasma Creatinine Ratio?

Nephrologists seem to love ratios. The urinary albumin-to-creatinine ratio (UACR) and the urinary protein-to-creatinine ratio (UPCR) are discussed in Chapter 4. And fractional excretions, discussed in Chapter 3, are essentially a ratio of ratios, that is, the ratio of the urine-to-plasma concentration ratio of the substance of interest to the urine-to-plasma creatinine concentration ratio.

What about the urine-to-plasma creatinine ratio (U/P Cr)? It is the denominator of the fractional excretion of sodium (FENa) formula, so why do we need it if we have FENa? The reason is that the U/P Cr is a measure of water reabsorption/excretion whereas FENa reflects sodium reabsorption/excretion. Also sometimes you may have only a urine creatinine (UCr) but no urine sodium (UNa), since someone has ordered a UACR or UPCR.

Most healthy individuals are in an antidiuretic state most of the time (so they are not spending too much time going to the bathroom!). A U/P Cr of 100/1 is thus typical. How is the kidney able to concentrate creatinine 100-fold? There are only two possible ways that the kidney could accomplish this task. Either it could be secreting creatinine against a huge concentration gradient (which does not happen!) or it is reabsorbing 99% of the filtered water (which does happen). Many trainees initially suggest the first mechanism and not the correct one when asked this question.

Here is another more colloquial way to teach the concept. Your grandmother asks you to make her a pot of tea. You do so, but after she pours herself a cup and takes one sip, she returns the pot to you and states,

"This tastes like water—make it 100 times stronger!" Now you could add 100 times more tea to the pot, but there is no more tea in the house. So instead you boil off 99% of the water, which makes grandmother happy again (albeit with a much smaller cup of tea).

Some like to convert the U/P Cr to fractional excretion of water (FEH_2O).

$$FEH_2O = H_2O \text{ excreted}/H_2O \text{ filtered} = \text{Urine flow/GFR} = V/GFR = V/[(UCr \times V)/PCr] = P/U \text{ Cr} \times 100$$

So, if the U/P Cr is 100, the P/U Cr is 0.01 and FEH_2O is 1%, which is the same thing as saying that 99% of the water has been reabsorbed. If the U/P Cr is 40, the FEH_2O is 2.5% or 97.5% of the water has been reabsorbed.

Let us take the example of a healthy male medical student weighing 72 kg who excretes 20 mg/kg of creatinine in the urine in 24 hours. His 24-hour UCr excretion is thus 1,440 mg. If he makes 1,440 mL of urine a day, his UCr concentration will be 100 mg/dL. Assuming his serum creatinine is 1 mg/dL, he will have a U/P Cr of 100/1 or FEH_2O of 1%. Now let us assume that he has a big test coming up and has to study for 24 hours straight and has no time to eat or drink. He is now in a marked antidiuretic state and his daily urine volume has decreased to 720 mL. If his serum creatinine is still 1 mg/dL, his U/P Cr will be 200/1 or FEH_2O of 0.5%. After the big test, he goes on a 24-hour drinking binge at the local pub. His urine volume now quadruples to 5,760 mL/24 hours. Now his U/P Cr is 25/1 or FEH_2O of 4%.

TABLE 5.1 Urinary Tests in Prerenal Failure versus Acute Tubular Injury

Laboratory Test	Prerenal Failure	Acute Tubular Injury
Urine sodium (mEq/L)	<20	>40
Urine osmolality (mmol/kg)	>350	~300
Urine-to-plasma creatinine (U/P Cr)	>40	<20
Laboratory Test	**Prerenal Failure**	**Acute Tubular Injury**
Fractional excretion of sodium (FENa) (%)	<1	>1(2)
Fractional excretion of urea (FEurea) (%)	<35	>50
Urine sediment	Hyaline casts	Pigmented granular casts ("muddy-brown casts")

This is all fine, but how does U/P Cr or FEH$_2$O help in clinical practice? Just as FENa is useful in the differential diagnosis of acute renal failure, FEH$_2$O is also useful. The higher the U/P Cr and lower the FEH$_2$O, the more likely the patient is in prerenal failure and has intact tubular function (see Chapter 9). Diagnostic urine tests that have been used in the differential diagnosis of acute renal failure are shown in Table 5.1 (Handa and Morrin, 1967; Miller et al., 1978). Naturally, there is a "gray zone" as these disorders are not mutually exclusive.

PATIENT 1

A 60-year-old male smoker with hypertension and severe peripheral vascular disease is admitted for dyspnea. One week previously he had been started on an angiotensin-converting enzyme (ACE) inhibitor, after which he noted a marked decrease in urine output followed by leg swelling and progressive shortness of breath. His serum creatinine, which was 1.6 mg/dL when measured a month ago is now 4 mg/dL. On examination, he is hypertensive and has bibasilar rales and edema. There is an audible epigastric bruit and bilateral femoral bruits. His U/P Cr is 400/1.

Q: What is the etiology of acute renal failure?

A: First, a word on semantics. The rapid development of renal failure is now commonly called acute kidney injury (AKI), rather than acute renal failure. Although this patient assuredly has acute kidney disease (AKD), the term AKD is not in widespread use, though very logical. Although the senior medical resident and attending called this AKI of uncertain etiology, an astute medical student recognized that the history, physical, and laboratory findings were highly suggestive of bilateral renal artery stenosis. In this setting, administration of any renin–angiotensin system (RAS) blocker will dilate efferent arterioles and may cause a marked decline in GFR. The kidneys stay well perfused however, and there is generally no ischemic injury (thus the term AKI does not fit well here). Stopping the ACE inhibitor resulted in improvement of renal function. A subsequent renal angiogram confirmed high-grade bilateral renal artery stenosis with an atrophic right kidney. He underwent angioplasty and stent placement of the left renal artery, which resulted in better blood pressure control and normalization of renal function.

PATIENT 2

A 75-year-old woman with chronic obstructive lung disease (COPD) is admitted with fever and alteration of mental status. On examination, she appears volume depleted with hypotension, flat neck veins, decreased skin turgor, and no edema. She is not taking diuretics and has had no vomiting or diarrhea. Her serum creatinine is 2 mg/dL (baseline 1 month previously was 0.5 mg/dL). She is diagnosed with "prerenal AKI" by the house staff and is started on intravenous fluids. The medical student assigned to the case reviews the urinary indices, which reveal a FENa of 2.5%. The actual data are as follows:

$$FENa = [(UNa/PNa)/(UCr/PCr)] \times 100 = [(35/140)/(20/2)] \times 100 = (0.25/10) \times 100 = 2.5\%$$

Q: What is the etiology of acute renal failure?

A: The student noted that the U/P Cr was 10/1 and thus the renal tubules were only reabsorbing 90% of the filtered water (despite reabsorbing 97.5% of the filtered sodium). He diagnosed acute tubular injury and predicted that renal failure would become more severe in the coming days. His prediction proved to be correct, as the patient did not respond to intravenous fluids and ultimately required dialysis.

References

Handa SP, Morrin PA. Diagnostic indices in acute renal failure. *Can Med Assoc J.* 1967;96:78–82.
Miller TR, Anderson RJ, Linas SL, et al. Urinary diagnostic indices in acute renal failure: a prospective study. *Ann Intern Med.* 1978;89(1):47–50.

6

Is It Helpful to Diagnose a Triple Acid–Base Disturbance? (Or Is It Just a Mental Exercise?)

If nephrologists love ratios, they get absolutely ecstatic over complex acid–base disturbances. Back in the days, the mettle of a nephrology attending was indicated by how well he (or she) could solve a complex electrolyte or acid–base disorder "on the fly." Dr. Donald Seldin from Southwestern in Dallas was famous for his ability to teach "metabolic alkalosis" using "Socratic methods" to keep his audience focused!

The basic steps in acid–base analysis are straightforward, providing an orderly, logical plan is followed. An arterial blood gas (ABG) is necessary for definitive acid–base analysis.

These are the steps to follow:

1. Look at pH to determine if there is acidemia (pH <7.38) or alkalemia (pH >7.46)
   - If pH is low, there must be a primary acidosis.
   - If pH is high, there must be a primary alkalosis.
2. Look at HCO_3^- and PCO_2 to determine the type of acidosis or alkalosis present
   - $[HCO_3^-]$ is low in metabolic acidosis and high in metabolic alkalosis.
   - PCO_2 is low in respiratory alkalosis and high in respiratory acidosis.

   At this point, the primary acid–base process should be evident, that is, metabolic or respiratory acidosis or alkalosis.
3. Determine if compensation (adaptation) is appropriate

   Henderson's equation shows the relationship between pH, PCO_2, and HCO_3^-:

$$[H^+] = (24 \times PCO_2)/[HCO_3^-]$$

39

From this formula, it is evident that in order to maintain $[H^+]$ near-normal, a primary change in either $[HCO_3^-]$ or Pco_2 should result in a counterbalancing change of the other in the same direction, that is,

- Metabolic acidosis is compensated by respiratory alkalosis (hyperventilation).
- Metabolic alkalosis is compensated by respiratory acidosis (hypoventilation).
- Chronic respiratory acidosis is compensated by metabolic alkalosis.
- Chronic respiratory alkalosis is compensated by metabolic acidosis.
- There is little adaptation to acute respiratory acidosis or alkalosis because it requires 24 to 48 hours for the kidneys to adapt to a primary respiratory disorder.

The expected compensations (adaptations) to primary acid–base disturbances have been determined empirically and are given in Table 6.1 (Bushinsky et al., 1982; Emmett, 2006).

When compensation is less or greater than expected, this suggests the presence of another primary disorder. For instance, in metabolic acidosis, if Pco_2 is higher than expected from Table 6.1, there is evidence for a coexisting primary respiratory acidosis (even though the Pco_2 may still be below the normal range). Another helpful thing to keep in mind: with a simple acid–base disturbance, the pH will rarely be in the normal range, as compensation for a primary disturbance is not "complete," that is, normal pH is not completely restored. Either a normal pH or a very abnormal pH is frequently seen in double acid–base disorders. A normal pH can occur if the extent of acidosis is balanced by a similar extent of alkalosis. However, if both types of

TABLE 6.1   Expected Compensation for Primary Acid–Base Disorders

Type	Primary Change	Secondary Adaptation
Metabolic acidosis	Decrease in $[HCO_3^-]$ of 1 mEq/L	Decrease in Pco_2 of 1.2 mm Hg
Metabolic alkalosis	Increase in $[HCO_3^-]$ of 1 mEq/L	Increase in Pco_2 of 0.7 mm Hg
Respiratory acidosis	Increase in Pco_2 of 10 mm Hg	Acute: Increase in $[HCO_3^-]$ of 1 mEq/L Chronic: Increase in $[HCO_3^-]$ of 3.5 mEq/L
Respiratory alkalosis	Decrease in Pco_2 of 10 mm Hg	Acute: Decrease in $[HCO_3^-]$ of 2 mEq/L Chronic: Decrease in $[HCO_3^-]$ of 4–5 mEq/L

acidosis or both types of alkalosis coexist, the pH may be very low or very high, respectively.

4. Calculate anion gap

The anion gap (AG) is the difference between the plasma concentration of sodium—the major extracellular cation—and the sum of the concentrations of the major extracellular anions chloride and bicarbonate, that is, $[Na^+] - ([Cl^-] + [HCO_3^-])$. Stated differently, the "AG" occurs due to a higher concentration of unmeasured anions (i.e., not chloride or bicarbonate) than unmeasured cations (i.e., not sodium). The normal AG (NAG) is about 10 to 14 mEq/L (Fig. 6.1). Note: HCO_3^- (calculated from pH and Pco_2 on an ABG) is very similar to total CO_2 (bicarbonate plus dissolved CO_2, as measured in the chemistry laboratory). For clinical purposes, they can generally be taken to be equivalent. Since an ABG is not always available, total CO_2 is conventionally used to calculate AG, though technically this is not correct as total CO_2 includes a small amount of uncharged CO_2.

If the AG is >20 mEq/L, there is an AG metabolic acidosis (lesser elevations are less specific), but keep in mind that albumin is an anion, so severe hypoalbuminemia will lower the AG (by ~2.5 mEq/L for each decrement of 1 g/dL of serum albumin). Theoretically, one

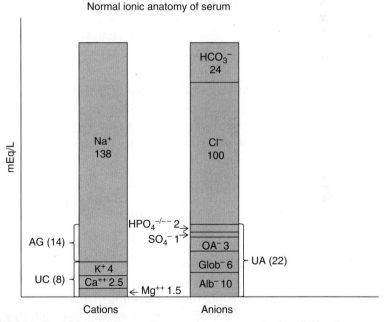

FIGURE 6.1 The AG is the difference between the unmeasured anions (UA) and unmeasured cations (UC). OA, organic acids; Glob, globulin; Alb, albumin.

would expect that, in a high AG (HAG) acidosis, for every millimole (or milliequivalent) of bicarbonate titrated by H^+, there would be one millimole (or milliequivalent) of retained anion. This supposition leads to the "delta–delta" concept (also known as "bicarbonate gap"). If the change in (delta) bicarbonate is greater than the change in (delta) AG, this suggests a combined HAG/NAG acidosis. If delta AG is much greater than delta bicarbonate, this suggests the presence of a metabolic alkalosis that is independently increasing bicarbonate levels ("hidden" metabolic alkalosis). It should be pointed out that this latter supposition may not always be true, as with more severe degrees of AG acidosis, buffers other than bicarbonate are also utilized to titrate H^+, and thus "delta AG" will be greater than "delta bicarbonate." Unless metabolic acidosis is severe, the delta–delta concept works fairly well in practice though has limitations (Rashtegar, 2007). The AG should be corrected for the serum albumin concentration when using the delta–delta analysis.

HAG metabolic acidosis can occur from either an increase in organic acid production, such as in lactic acidosis or ketoacidosis, or from the retention of phosphoric and sulfuric acids in renal failure. NAG acidosis is usually caused by either diarrhea or renal disease (renal tubular acidosis [RTA] or chronic kidney disease [CKD]). Alkalosis can cause a slight increase in AG (<20 mEq/L) due to increased lactic acid formation.

PATIENT 1

A 55-year-old woman with known CKD presents to the ER with decreased appetite, nausea, and vomiting. She was told several months previously that she would need to start dialysis soon but got scared and did not return to clinic. Blood chemistries reveal (in mmol/L) the following:

Na^+ 138	ABG:
K^+ 4	pH 7.40
Cl^- 90	Pco_2 40 mm Hg
Total CO_2 24	HCO_3^- 24 mEq/L

Q: What is the acid–base disturbance?

A: A quick glance at the data might be misleading in this case. The ABG values are completely normal. Remember however that a normal pH is consistent with either no acid–base disorder or a mixed disorder where there is both an acidosis and an alkalosis. Also remember to always calculate the AG, which in this case is $138 - (90 + 24) = 24$ mEq/L, indicating the presence of an AG acidosis. This patient thus has a double acid–base disturbance, both an AG acidosis from uremia and a metabolic alkalosis from vomiting. It just happened that they balanced each other out so that all of her laboratory values (except the blood chloride) are normal.

PATIENT 2

A 55-year-old man presents to the ER with stomach pain. He denies vomiting. On examination, he is no distress but is noted to be hyperventilating. His serum chemistries reveal (in mmol/L) the following:

Na^+ 140	ABG:
K^+ 2.6	pH 7.86
Cl^- 69	Pco_2 23 mm Hg
Total CO_2 40	HCO_3^- 40 mEq/L

Q1: What is the acid–base disorder?

A1: This might appear at first glance to be another double acid–base disturbance; unlike the first case, in which there was a counterbalancing acidosis and alkalosis leading to a normal pH, in this case there is profound alkalemia due to the presence of both metabolic and respiratory alkalosis. However, remember to always calculate the AG! In this case, the AG is $140 - (69 + 40) = 31$ mEq/L. Therefore, despite a pH of 7.86, the patient has a concomitant HAG metabolic acidosis, and thus a triple disturbance!

Q2: What is the etiology?

A2: As it turns out, the realization that this patient had a triple acid–base disturbance was key to the correct diagnosis. A salicylate level was in the toxic range. Salicylism causes both HAG metabolic acidosis (primarily due to lactic acidosis) and primary respiratory alkalosis (due to drug-induced stimulation of the respiratory center). What about the metabolic alkalosis? Upon further questioning, the patient admitted to taking high-dose Alka-Seltzer to treat his pain. Alka-Seltzer contains bicarbonate as well as salicylate.

References

Bushinsky DA, Coe FL, Katzenberg C, et al. Arterial Pco_2 in chronic metabolic acidosis. *Kidney Int.* 1982;22(3):311–314.

Emmett M. Anion-gap interpretation: the old and the new. *Nat Clin Pract Nephrol.* 2006;2(1):4–5.

Rashtegar A. Use of the $\Delta AG/\Delta HCO_3^-$ ratio in the diagnosis of mixed acid–base disorders. *J Am Soc Nephrol.* 2007;18:2429–2431.

7

Why Are Disorders of Sodium Concentration So Difficult?

There are two important reasons why sodium concentration disorders (dysnatremias) are challenging. First, making the correct clinical diagnosis can be difficult. Second, the correct treatment regimen in acutely symptomatic patients is a high-stakes issue, as incorrect treatment can lead to a catastrophic outcome. With acute symptomatic hyponatremia, failure to rapidly raise the plasma sodium in a patient with cerebral edema may result in permanent brain damage or even herniation and death, whereas raising the plasma sodium too much may cause permanent brain damage due to the development of osmotic demyelination syndrome (ODS). In the 1980s, there was a controversy in the literature and a series of debates at nephrology meetings, with Allen Arieff on the side of rapid correction (Arieff, 1986) and Richard Sterns preaching caution (Sterns et al., 1986). Robert Narins wondered if it was really true that "haste made waste" (Narins, 1986). Actually, both sides can be correct, depending on the situation. In the rare patient with acute symptomatic hyponatremia (occurring within minutes to hours), rapid correction is necessary to treat brain edema. In most patients, however, even symptomatic hyponatremia is chronic (>48 hours in duration), and caution is advised. A 1989 article by Sterns "The Treatment of Hyponatremia: Unsafe at Any Speed?" followed by his 1990 article "The Treatment of Hyponatremia: First, Do No Harm," and a 1990 discussion by Tomas Berl "Treating Hyponatremia: Damned If We Do and Damned If We Don't" pointed out that the brain is encased in a skull and thus there is a limit to the amount of brain edema that can occur without leading to herniation and death (Sterns, 1989, 1990; Berl, 1990). Brain water content therefore cannot exceed about 10% above normal. Thus, it follows that if symptoms are due to cerebral edema, they should be corrected by an increase in serum sodium of 10% or less regardless of the severity of hyponatremia.

It is of interest that we seem to have come full circle in our views on management of acute symptomatic hyponatremia. In the first edition of Harrison's *Principles of Internal Medicine*, published in 1950, it was recommended that patients with symptomatic water intoxication promptly receive hypertonic saline to increase the plasma sodium by about 2 to 6 mmol/L. Currently, marathon runners with acute symptomatic hyponatremia due to water intoxication are treated in a similar fashion (Hew-Butler et al., 2008); most authorities today favor rapid correction of up to 6 mmol/L in severely symptomatic patients and to avoid an increase in plasma sodium of more than 8 mmol/L in the first 24 hours (Sterns, 2014). Such a regimen should provide the benefit of treating cerebral edema while minimizing the chance of the later development of ODS.

PATHOGENESIS OF HYPONATREMIA

We will now address the pathogenesis of hyponatremia. On occasion, the plasma sodium concentration [Na] may be artifactually low, that is, pseudohyponatremia. In such cases, the plasma osmolality is normal rather than low as would be expected. This used to be rather commonly observed in the presence of hyperglobulinemia (such as myeloma) or marked hypertriglyceridemia. Fortunately, this now rarely occurs with modern laboratory methods, except at extremes of globulin or triglyceride concentrations, and further discussion will be focused on true hyponatremia. Patients with high plasma concentrations of an osmotically active substance (usually glucose, but sometimes mannitol or other substances) can develop hyperosmolal hyponatremia due to shift of water from the intracellular (ICF) to extracellular fluid (ECF). Most patients with hyponatremia, however, have hypoosmolal hyponatremia.

In true hyponatremic states, the plasma [Na] reflects the relative amount of sodium to water in the plasma, but does not give any information about the absolute amount of either, which must be determined clinically. Thus, the clinician must determine the meaning of the plasma [Na] in the context of the patient's clinical picture, and in particular the volume status. Therefore, we classify hypoosmolal hyponatremic patients as being hypovolemic, euvolemic, or hypervolemic, depending on the clinically perceived assessment of ECF volume (Table 7.1). If a patient has no edema, flat neck veins, and an orthostatic fall in blood pressure (with an increase in heart rate), this is a fairly reliable indication of volume depletion. If there is edema, this is good evidence for ECF excess or

TABLE 7.1	Causes of Hypoosmolar Hyponatremia			
Hypovolemic		**Euvolemic**	**Hypervolemic**	
FENa <1; Uosm > Posm	FENa >1; Uosm ~ or > Posm	FENa usually >1; Uosm > Posm except < Posm in reset osmostat, psychogenic polydipsia, and beer drinker's syndrome	FENa <1; Uosm > Posm	FENa >1; Uosm ~ Posm
GI or sweat losses	Salt-losing nephropathy	SIADH/Reset osmostat/ NSIAD	CHF	Renal failure
	Adrenal insufficiency/ isolated	Psychogenic polydipsia	Cirrhosis	
	Mineralocorticoid deficiency	Beer drinker's syndrome	Nephrotic syndrome	
	Diuretics	Exercise hyponatremia Postoperative hyponatremia		
		Drugs either stimulating ADH secretion or increasing its action		

FENa, fractional excretion of sodium; Uosm, urine osmolality; Posm, plasma osmolality; GI, gastrointestinal; NSIAD, nephrogenic syndrome of inappropriate antidiuresis; ADH, antidiuretic hormone; CHF, congestive heart failure.
From Moinuddin IK, Leehey DJ. *Handbook of Nephrology.* Philadelphia, PA: Lippincott Williams & Wilkins; 2013.

hypervolemia. If neither is present, we say that the patient is euvolemic. However, it is not always easy to determine ECF volume status at the bedside. In some situations (e.g., severe hypoalbuminemia, inferior vena cava compression), edema may be due to alteration in Starling forces (i.e., the ECF, which is usually distributed in an approximately 1:3 ratio between plasma and interstitial fluid, is now preferentially distributed in the interstitial space compared to the plasma). Such patients may actually be plasma-volume depleted despite having edema. This is not at all uncommon in the ICU setting. Moreover, despite edema, many patients have a decrease in what has been termed "effective blood volume," meaning that even though the ECF is expanded, there is activation of neurohormonal pathways that signal the kidneys that effective volume is low and to conserve salt and water. Common examples are congestive heart failure (where low cardiac output is perceived as low effective volume) and liver cirrhosis (where systemic vasodilatation is perceived as low effective volume) despite the presence of ascites and/or edema. In all of these conditions, hyponatremia will be present if there is a relatively greater increase in total body water (TBW) relative to total body sodium (TBNa).

To add additional difficulty, we also need to be concerned about potassium in addition to sodium and water when we are analyzing sodium problems. Why? The answer lies in the fact that whereas sodium is essentially confined to the ECF, potassium is mostly in the ICF. Administration of sodium will increase the content of sodium in the ECF; the increase in ECF [Na] will then draw water out of the ICF by osmosis. The change in plasma [Na] will thus depend on the amount of sodium administered and the sum of ECF and ICF volume, that is, TBW. On the other hand, administration of potassium will increase the content of potassium in the ICF; the increase in ICF [K] will draw water into the cells, thus increasing the plasma [Na].

Since ECF [Na] is approximately equal to ICF [K]:

$$\text{Plasma [Na]} = (\text{TBNa} + \text{TBK})/\text{TBW}$$

Plasma [Na] thus reflects the relationship between total body cations (sodium plus potassium) and TBW. This concept was first proposed and provided experimental evidence by Edelman and colleagues in 1958. Edelman's formula was a bit more complex since not all sodium in the body is osmotically active, but the simpler formula works well in clinical practice.

Administration of water will lead to a decrease in plasma [Na]. In a healthy individual, a very small (~1%) decrease in plasma sodium or osmolality will inhibit antidiuretic hormone secretion with resultant water diuresis, serving to normalize the plasma [Na]. Thus, with rare exceptions, hypoosmolal hyponatremia is due to impaired renal water excretion.

Assuming there has not been time for renal water excretion to occur or there is a pronounced defect in renal water excretion, how does one calculate the predicted change in plasma [Na$^+$] with addition of water to the body?

Using a formula derived from Avogadro's law:

$$V_1 \times C_1 = V_2 \times C_2$$

where V_1 = initial TBW; V_2 = final TBW; C_1 = initial plasma [Na]; and C_2 = final plasma [Na].

The TBW is generally estimated as 0.6 × body weight (kg) in men (0.5 × body weight in women). In a 70-kg male patient, the TBW would thus be 42 L. If the initial plasma [Na] is 140 mmol/L, and 3 L of water is added to the body (with no water losses), the TBW is now 45 L.

Therefore,

$$\text{Final plasma [Na]} = (\text{Initial TBW} \times \text{Initial plasma [Na]})/\text{Final TBW}$$
$$= (42 \times 140)/45 = 131 \text{ mmol/L}$$

What if 100 mmol of sodium is added to the body? Administered sodium will enter and stay in the ECF (assuming no excretion). TBW has been classically stated to be one-third in the ECF and two-thirds in the ICF (although 45% and 55%, respectively, have more recently been shown to be typical). For our purposes, we will stick to the 1/3:2/3 ratio. In this case, TBNa before sodium is added is:

$$140 \text{ mmol/L} \times 14 \text{ L} = 1,960 \text{ mmol}$$

After addition of 100 mmol sodium, one might think that there is now 2,060 mmol sodium distributed in 14 L, which would result in a final plasma [Na] of 2,060/14 = 147 mmol/L. However, due to the increase in ECF osmolality, water will move from the ICF to the ECF, and the final plasma [Na] will actually be less (~142 mmol/L).

What if 100 mmol of potassium is added to the body? Administered potassium will enter and stay in the ICF (assuming no excretion). In this case, TBK before potassium is added is:

$$140 \text{ mmol/L} \times 28 \text{ L} = 3,920 \text{ mmol}$$

After addition of 100 mmol potassium, due to the increased ICF osmolality, water will move from the ECF to the ICF, thus also raising the plasma [Na$^+$] to about 142 mmol/L.

According to the modified Edelman equation:

$$\text{Plasma [Na]} = (\text{TBNa} + \text{TBK})/\text{TBW}$$

$$\text{TBNa} + \text{TBK} = 140 \text{ mmol/L} \times 42 \text{ L} = 5,880 \text{ mmol}$$

Addition of either 100 mmol of sodium or potassium will have identical effects on plasma [Na$^+$], that is, raise it to (5,880 + 100)/42 L = 142 mmol/L.

The above examples assume no loss of either sodium or potassium from the body. In most patients, there will be loss of electrolytes, predominantly in the urine but also in stool, sweat, and sometimes via surgical drains. In most patients, we need to be concerned only with urinary losses, and one can use urinary electrolyte losses to predict changes in plasma [Na].

For instance, let us assume that a patient makes 2 L of urine with a urine [Na + K] of 70 mmol/L. One can think of this as the loss of 1 L of electrolyte-free water and 1 L of water containing a [Na + K] of 140 mmol/L. The 1 L of electrolyte-free water loss will raise the plasma [Na$^+$] to:

$$\text{Final plasma [Na]} = (\text{Initial TBW} \times \text{Initial plasma [Na]})/\text{Final TBW}$$
$$= (42 \times 140)/41 = 143 \text{ mmol/L}$$

Adrogué and Madias (2012) have published simple formulae that will predict the effect on plasma [Na$^+$] of either gain or loss of 1 L of fluid having any [Na + K]. They have used the terms *infusate formula* and *fluid loss formula*.

Infusate formula:

$$\text{Change in plasma [Na]} = (\text{Infusate [Na + K]} - \text{Plasma [Na]})/(\text{TBW} + 1)$$

Fluid loss formula:

$$\text{Change in plasma [Na]} = (\text{Plasma [Na]} - \text{Fluid [Na + K]})/(\text{TBW} - 1)$$

We will utilize these formulae in the case studies that follow.

Acute Hyponatremia

How should you treat a plasma [Na] of 110 mmol/L in a 70 kg postoperative male patient with seizures and coma? He is clinically euvolemic. We will assume TBW in this male patient to be 0.6 × body weight, that is, 42 L.

Since this is an emergency, the goal is to rapidly increase plasma [Na$^+$]. We will thus use 3% saline (513 mmol/L). Although administered sodium will stay in the ECF, the resultant increase in osmolality of the ECF will lead to a shift of fluid from the ICF to the ECF; thus, as discussed earlier, we think of the sodium distributing into the TBW.

$$\text{TBNa} + \text{TBK} = 110 \text{ mmol/L} \times 42 \text{ L} = 4,620 \text{ mmol}$$

Addition of 100 mL of 3% saline (51 mmol of sodium in 100 mL) will raise plasma [Na] to (4,620 + 51)/42.1 L = 111 mmol/L.

Some prefer to use the "infusate formula," which will project the effect of 1 L of any infusate on plasma [Na]. This formula has the advantage that it will take into account the effect of any administered potassium, as administration of potassium will also increase plasma [Na]. The infusate formula will predict in this case as follows:

$$\text{Change in plasma [Na]} = (\text{Infusate [Na + K]} - \text{Plasma [Na]})/(\text{TBW} + 1)$$
$$= (513 - 110)/43 = 9.4 \text{ mmol/L}$$

It can be seen that approximately 200 to 600 mL of 3% saline will be necessary to increase the plasma [Na] by 2% to 6%.

PATIENT 2
Chronic Hypovolemic Hyponatremia

How should you treat a plasma [Na] of 110 mmol/L in a clinically hypovolemic but otherwise asymptomatic 60-kg female patient? We will assume TBW in this female patient to be 0.5 × body weight, that is, 30 L, and for now disregard any effect of urinary losses of electrolytes and water.

In this case, the goal is to avoid correcting plasma [Na$^+$] by more than 0.5 mmol/L/h or to more than 120 mmol/L in about 24 hours. We will use 0.9% saline (154 mmol/L).

$$\text{TBNa} + \text{TBK} = 110 \text{ mmol/L} \times 30 \text{ L} = 3{,}300 \text{ mmol}$$

Addition of 154 mmol of sodium in 1 L will raise plasma [Na$^+$] to (3,300 + 154)/31 L = 111.4 mmol/L.

The infusate formula will predict in this case as follows:

$$\begin{aligned}\text{Change in plasma [Na]} &= (\text{Infusate [Na + K]} \\ &\quad - \text{Plasma [Na]})/(\text{TBW} + 1) \\ &= (154 - 110)/31 = 1.4 \text{ mmol/L}\end{aligned}$$

One can see that in the absence of urinary or other water losses, the change in plasma [Na] would be minimal. However, unless the patient has no renal function, this is not the case in reality (see later).

PATIENT 3
Chronic Euvolemic Hyponatremia

How should you treat a plasma [Na] of 110 mmol/L in a clinically euvolemic asymptomatic 60-kg female patient with a presumptive diagnosis of SIADH (syndrome of inappropriate antidiuretic hormone)? We will again assume TBW in this female patient to be 0.5 × body weight, that is, 30 L.

Even though this patient is clinically euvolemic, that is, ECF volume appears to be normal, plasma volume is expanded due to renal water retention. In this case, what you want to do is remove water. This can be accomplished by fluid restriction alone. Administration of a loop diuretic such as furosemide to increase water loss into the urine will speed up the process, but electrolyte losses will need to be replaced. A more elegant option would be to give tolvaptan, which blocks the V_2 receptor and will cause water diuresis but not natriuresis, though this is rarely necessary (and is very expensive).

How much negative fluid balance needs to be achieved?

Initial TBW $\times$ Initial plasma [Na] = Final TBW $\times$ Final plasma [Na]

This becomes

$$30 \times 110 = V_2 \times 120$$

$$V_2 = (30 \times 110)/120 = 27.5$$

Therefore, a negative water balance of 2.5 L will be needed.

The previous three examples were all oversimplified as they did not consider the effects of urinary electrolyte and water loss. In reality, they are important. For instance, in hypovolemic and euvolemic hyponatremia, the effect of saline administration on plasma [Na] is affected by any concomitant urinary electrolyte and water losses. Thus, one needs to consider the urine–plasma electrolyte ratio, that is, urine [Na + K]/plasma [Na]. (We do not worry about plasma [K], as it is quantitatively small.) If administration of 1 L of isotonic saline (154 mmol/L) is accompanied by excretion of 1 L of urine with a [Na + K] of 154 mmol/L, we would expect no change in plasma [Na]. If urine [Na + K] is <154, plasma [Na] will increase and if urine [Na + K] is >154, plasma [Na] will actually decrease. (The former is typical of hypovolemic hyponatremia, but the latter can occur in some cases of euvolemic hyponatremia due to SIADH.)

In reality, volume expansion in the patient in Case Study 3 will likely lead to an increase in urinary electrolyte loss such that urine [Na + K] > plasma [Na], with resultant worsening of hyponatremia. Therefore, a reasonable approach is to fluid restrict the patient and administer furosemide with the goal to correct plasma [Na] to 120 mmol/L over 24 hours. Let us assume that after administration of furosemide, urine [Na + K] = 75 mmol/L. If we also assume insensible water loss of 700 mL a day and fluid restriction to 700 mL a day, the expected change in plasma [Na] for each liter of urine lost will be predicted by the "fluid loss formula."

$$\begin{aligned} \text{Change in plasma [Na]} &= (\text{Plasma [Na]} - \text{Urine [Na + K]})/(\text{TBW} - 1) \\ &= (110 - 75)/29 = 1.2 \text{ mmol/L} \end{aligned}$$

It can be seen that the patient would need to excrete about 8 L of urine with the aforementioned electrolyte composition to achieve the desired change in plasma [Na]. Administration of sodium and potassium will replace urinary electrolyte losses and lead to more rapid correction of hyponatremia.

Let us assume the patient consumes a diet containing 200 mmol of sodium plus potassium during the initial 24-hour period. The effect on plasma [Na] is predicted by the modified Edelman formula:

$$\text{Plasma [Na]} = (\text{TBNa} + \text{TBK})/\text{TBW}$$

In this case,

$$110 = 3{,}300/30$$

Administration of 200 mmol of sodium plus potassium will lead to 117 = 3,500/30, or a 7 mmol/L increase in plasma $[Na^+]$. So now the patient needs to lose only about 3 L of urine in order for the plasma [Na] to correct to 120 mmol/L.

Another approach is not to rely solely upon diet (as the patient may not be eating well), but to administer sodium chloride (salt) tablets. A 1-g salt tablet contains 1,000 mg/(58.5 mg/mmol) = 17 mmol sodium chloride and thus 17 mmol sodium. Administration of six tablets daily will provide about 100 mmol sodium, so now the patient would have to consume only 100 mmol of sodium plus potassium in the diet.

PATIENT 4
Chronic Hypervolemic Hyponatremia

How should you treat a plasma [Na] of 110 mmol/L in a clinically hypervolemic (edematous) but otherwise asymptomatic 60-kg female patient?

The goal again is to increase plasma [Na] by 0.5 mmol/L/h to 120 mmol/L in about 24 hours.

Using the same Avogadro formula as in Case Study 3, we will need to achieve a negative water balance of 2.5 L.

In this case, we will use furosemide, as we want to get rid of both salt and water. Since furosemide leads to loss of electrolytes in the urine, it is again essential to consider urinary losses.

Let us assume the patient excretes 1 L of urine with a [Na + K] of 60 mmol/L after administration of furosemide. The expected increase in plasma [Na] per liter of urine excreted can be estimated by the "fluid loss formula," that is,

$$\text{Change in plasma [Na]} = (\text{Plasma [Na]} - \text{Urine [Na + K]})/(\text{TBW} - 1)$$
$$= (110 - 60)/29 = 1.7 \text{ mmol/L}$$

Therefore, excretion of about 6 L of urine will affect a 10-mmol/L rise in plasma [Na].

In this case, a high sodium diet is not indicated, as the patient is edematous, but replacement of urinary potassium losses is indicated and will also help correct the hyponatremia.

PATIENT 5

Chronic Hypovolemic Hyponatremia Accompanied by Hypokalemia

How should you treat a plasma [Na] of 110 mmol/L in a clinically hypovolemic 60-kg female patient who also has severe hypokalemia (plasma [K] 2 mmol/L)? This situation is not uncommon in patients with renal or extrarenal fluid losses. We will again assume TBW in this female patient to be 0.5 × body weight, that is, 30 L.

You decide to treat the patient with isotonic saline containing 40 mmol/L of K^+ at a rate of 250 mL/h. In this case, we need to use the "infusate formula" to predict the change in plasma [Na]:

$$\text{Change in plasma [Na]} = (\text{Infusate [Na + K]} - \text{Plasma [Na]})/(\text{TBW} + 1)$$
$$= (194 - 110)/31 = 2.7 \text{ mmol/L}$$

Therefore, at an IV infusion rate of 250 mL/h, we will predict a rate of correction of slightly more than 0.5 mmol/L/h.

In actuality, the plasma [Na] may rise even faster than this, as due to the hypovolemic state, we expect urine [Na + K] < plasma [Na]. Initially, urine flow rate is likely to be low, so electrolyte-free water losses in the urine are expected to be minimal, but a more rapid than expected correction of plasma [Na^+] may occur after volume repletion leads to an increase in renal water excretion. It will likely therefore be necessary to administer a solution with a lower sodium concentration or decrease the IV infusion rate.

PATIENT 6

Chronic Euvolemic Hyponatremia Accompanied by Hypokalemia

How should you treat a plasma [Na] of 110 mmol/L accompanied by a plasma [K] of 2 mmol/L in a clinically euvolemic but otherwise asymptomatic 60-kg female patient? This patient was recently started on a thiazide diuretic. We will again assume TBW in this female patient to be 0.5 × body weight, that is, 30 L.

In practice, such patients are often treated similarly to the patient in Case Study 5, that is, with isotonic saline containing 40 mmol/L of K, though at a slower rate (e.g., 125 mL/h). What is likely to happen?

The infusate formula will again predict the change in plasma [Na] as follows:

$$\text{Change in plasma [Na]} = (\text{Infusate [Na + K]} - \text{Plasma [Na]})/(\text{TBW} + 1)$$
$$= (194 - 110)/31 = 2.7 \text{ mmol/L}$$

This patient is likely to have large concentrations of electrolytes in the urine due to the effect of the thiazide, that is, urine [Na + K] ~ plasma [Na$^+$], which may increase further when volume is administered. Let us assume a urine [Na + K] of 180 mmol/L after volume administration.

The fluid loss formula will predict the change in plasma [Na] as follows:

$$\text{Change in plasma [Na]} = (\text{Plasma [Na]} - \text{Urine [Na + K]})/(\text{TBW} - 1)$$
$$= (110 - 180)/29 = -2.4 \text{ mmol/L}$$

The effects of the fluid infused and fluid loss will essentially cancel out and hyponatremia will not be improved.

What happens if we just give potassium and fluid restrict the patient? The effect of giving 40 mmol of oral K is as follows. Since we are not expanding the ECF volume (actually decreasing it a bit by shift of water into cells), additional natriuresis will not occur, and we will assume urine [Na + K] of 110 mmol/L.

Here, the infusate formula does not really apply, since we are not giving IV potassium. However, if the oral potassium is all absorbed and enters the ICF, we would predict the change in plasma [Na] as follows:

$$\text{Plasma [Na]} = (\text{TBNa} + \text{TBK})/\text{TBW}$$

$$\text{Change in plasma [Na]} = \text{Administered K/TBW} = 40/30 =$$
$$1.33 \text{ mmol/L}$$

The fluid loss formula will now predict the change in plasma [Na] as follows:

$$\text{Change in plasma [Na]} = (\text{Plasma [Na]} - \text{Urine [Na + K]})/(\text{TBW} - 1)$$
$$= (110 - 110)/29 = 0 \text{ mmol/L}$$

In this case, hyponatremia will be slightly improved.

Now let us shift our focus to hypernatremia. As with hyponatremia, the clinician must determine the meaning of the plasma [Na] in the context of the patient's clinical picture, and in particular the clinical estimation of ECF volume status. Therefore, we similarly classify hypernatremic patients as being hypovolemic, euvolemic, or hypervolemic (Table 7.2).

Causes of Hypernatremia		
Hypovolemic	**Euvolemic**	**Hypervolemic**
FENa <1; Uosm > Posm	FENa >1; Uosm ~ Posm	FENa usually <1; Uosm < Posm in DI; Uosm usually > Posm in other conditions	FENa >1; Uosm > Posm
GI or sweat losses	Osmotic diuresis Diuretics Postobstruction	DI Partial DI Nephrogenic DI	Primary aldosteronism Hypertonic fluids Salt-water drowning/ salt poisoning
	Salt-wasting nephropathy	Hypodipsia Respiratory or sweat (insensible) loss	

FENa, fractional excretion of sodium; Uosm, urine osmolality; Posm, plasma osmolality; GI, gastrointestinal; DI, diabetes insipidus
From Moinuddin IK, Leehey DJ. *Handbook of Nephrology.* Philadelphia, PA: Lippincott Williams & Wilkins; 2013.

The appropriate treatment will then be determined, with the caveat that acute hypernatremia is even more rare than acute hyponatremia, unless the patient drinks sea water or soy sauce (Carlberg et al., 2013) or is mistakenly given 5% saline rather than 5% dextrose (5% saline is no longer available in the United States for this reason). Since hypernatremia is virtually always chronic, there has been time for brain adaptation, and the rate of correction of plasma [Na] should not exceed 0.5 mmol/L/h.

PATIENT 7
Hypovolemic Hypernatremia

How should you treat a plasma [Na] of 160 mmol/L in a hypotensive clinically hypovolemic 60-kg female patient admitted from a nursing home? We will assume a TBW of 30 L (though it is undoubtedly lower due to volume depletion and dehydration).

Goal is to decrease plasma [Na] by about 0.5 mmol/L/h to 150 mmol/L in about 24 hours. We will use 0.9% saline, as in this case volume takes precedence over osmolality. Using the "infusate formula":

$$\text{Change in plasma [Na]} = (\text{Infusate [Na + K]} - \text{Plasma [Na]})/(\text{TBW} + 1)$$
$$= (154 - 160)/31 = -0.2 \text{ mmol/L}$$

Once hypotension is improved, we will switch to 0.45% saline. In this case,

Change in plasma [Na] = (Infusate [Na + K] − Plasma [Na])
$$/(TBW + 1) = (77 - 160)/31$$
$$= -2.7 \text{ mmol/L}$$

In order to avoid too rapid change in plasma [Na], we will limit the amount of 0.45% saline given to 3 L/day or less.

PATIENT 8
Euvolemic Hypernatremia

How should you treat a plasma [Na] of 160 mmol/L in an obtunded clinically euvolemic 60-kg female patient admitted from a nursing home? We will assume a TBW of 30 L (though it is likely lower due to dehydration).

Goal is to decrease plasma [Na] by 0.5 mmol/L/h to 150 mmol/L in about 24 hours. We will use D5W (5% dextrose in water).

Formula: Initial [Na] × Initial TBW = Desired [Na]
× Desired TBW

Therefore, Desired TBW = (Initial [Na] × Initial TBW)/Desired [Na]

Desired TBW = 160 mmol/L × 30 L/150 mmol/L
= 32 L; thus, 2 L of D5W is needed.

Plan: Give D5W at 83 mL/h × 24 h

A related method is to calculate a "free water deficit," which is equal to (desired TBW − initial TBW).

Desired Final TBW − Initial TBW
= {(Initial [Na] × Initial TBW)/Desired [Na]} − Initial TBW
= Initial TBW × {(Initial [Na]/Desired [Na]) − 1}

which in this case would be 30 L × [(160/150) − 1] = 2 L.

Let us see what happens when we use the "infusate formula."

Change in plasma [Na] = (Infusate [Na + K]
− Plasma [Na])/(TBW + 1)
$$= (0 - 160)/31 = -5.2 \text{ mmol/L}$$

In this case, the infusate formula gives a slightly higher estimate as it takes into account the water infused.

PATIENT 9

Hypervolemic Hypernatremia

How should you treat a plasma [Na] of 160 mmol/L in a 60-kg female ICU patient who has received large volumes of saline for the management of sepsis accompanied by acute kidney injury (AKI)? We will assume a TBW of 30 L (though it is actually higher due to volume overload).

Goal is to decrease plasma [Na] by 0.5 mmol/L/h to 150 mmol/L in about 24 hours. We will again use D5W.

Formula: Initial [Na] × Initial TBW = Desired [Na] × Desired TBW

Therefore, Desired TBW = (Initial [Na] × Initial TBW)/Desired [Na]

Desired TBW = (160 mmol/L × 30 L)/150 mmol/L
= 32 L; thus, 2 L of D5W is needed.

Plan: Give D5W at 83 mL/h × 24 h

Let us see what happens when we use the "infusate formula."

Change in plasma [Na] = (Infusate [Na + K]
− Plasma [Na])/(TBW + 1)
= (0 − 160)/31 = −5.2 mmol/L

So far this looks identical to Case Study 8. However, patients recovering from sepsis and AKI in the ICU often have copious water losses in the urine. Let us assume that this patient is excreting 4 L of urine daily with a urine [Na + K] of 80.

The fluid loss formula will predict the change in plasma [Na] as follows:

Change in plasma [Na] = (Plasma [Na]
− Urine [Na + K])/(TBW − 1)
= (160 − 80)/29 = 2.8 mmol/L

Thus, the plasma [Na] is predicted to increase by 11.2 mmol/L/day due to urinary water losses, which will balance the predicted decline from the administration of D5W. Correction of hypernatremia will require even more water to be administered, either intravenously or via the GI tract.

Important

All of the above examples are based on theoretical calculations. In real life, things change (in particular, urinary electrolyte losses can change with changing clinical status), so measure plasma and urine electrolytes frequently to guide therapy.

References

Adrogué HJ, Madias NE. The challenge of hyponatremia. *J Am Soc Nephrol.* 2012;23(7):1140–1148.

Arieff AI. Hyponatremia, convulsions, respiratory arrest, and permanent brain damage after elective surgery in healthy women. *N Engl J Med.* 1986;314(24):1529–1535.

Berl T. Treating hyponatremia: damned if we do and damned if we don't. *Kidney Int.* 1990;37(3):1006–1018.

Carlberg DJ, Borek HA, Syverud SA, et al. Survival of acute hypernatremia due to massive soy sauce ingestion. *J Emerg Med.* 2013;45(2):228–231.

Edelman IS, Liebman J, O'Meara MP, et al. Interrelations between serum sodium concentration, serum osmolarity and total exchangeable sodium, total exchangeable potassium and total body water. *J Clin Invest.* 1958;37(9):1236–1256.

Hew-Butler T, Ayus JC, Kipps C, et al. Statement of the Second International Exercise-Associated Hyponatremia Consensus Development Conference, New Zealand, 2007. *Clin J Sport Med.* 2008;18(2):111.

Narins RG. Therapy of hyponatremia: does haste make waste? *N Engl J Med.* 1986;314:1573–1575.

Sterns RH. The treatment of hyponatremia: unsafe at any speed? *Am Kidney Found Nephrol Lett.* 1989;6(1):1–10.

Sterns RH. The treatment of hyponatremia: first, do no harm. *Am J Med.* 1990;88:557–560.

Sterns RH. Overview of the treatment of hyponatremia in adults. Up-to-Date Website. http://www.uptodate.com/contents/overview-of-the-treatment-of-hyponatremia-in-adults. Accessed October 30, 2014.

Sterns RH, Riggs JE, Schochet SS Jr. Osmotic demyelination syndrome following correction of hyponatremia. *N Engl J Med.* 1986;314:1535–1542.

8

What Is Free Water Clearance and How Useful Is It?

Over 50 years ago, Homer Smith (1952) introduced the concept that the urine flow could be thought of as two separate compartments: one component containing osmotically active particles (osmoles) at the same concentration as that present in the plasma, and the other component consisting of either free water excreted (when the kidney is forming dilute urine) or free water reabsorbed (when the kidney is forming concentrated urine).

$$\text{Thus, } V = \text{Cosm} + \text{CH}_2\text{O}$$

where V is urine flow, Cosm is osmolal clearance, and CH_2O is free water clearance.

The volume of plasma that is cleared of osmoles per unit time (Cosm) $\times$ plasma osmolality (Posm) is equal to the urinary excretion of osmoles [urine osmolality (Uosm) $\times$ urine flow]. In mathematical form, it is as follows:

$$\text{Cosm} \times \text{Posm} = \text{Uosm} \times V$$

$$\text{Cosm} = \text{Uosm} \times V/\text{Posm}$$

Therefore,

$$\text{CH}_2\text{O} = V - \text{Cosm} = V - (\text{Uosm} \times V/\text{Posm})$$
$$= V(1 - \text{Uosm}/\text{Posm})$$

It can be readily seen that if urine is dilute, that is, Uosm $<$ Posm, free water clearance will be positive, and if urine is concentrated, that is, Uosm $>$ Posm, free water clearance will be negative (this means free water is being reabsorbed by the kidney). Observing the Uosm gives important qualitative information, but calculating free water clearance gives quantitative information.

Although free water clearance is a valid physiologic concept for the management of disorders of serum sodium concentration, it has been supplanted by the electrolyte-free water clearance (Goldberg, 1981).

Electrolyte-free water clearance (CeH_2O) means the clearance of water free of electrolytes (sodium, potassium, and accompanying anions) but not other solutes. Urine contains many other osmotically active particles, such as urea and ammonium, in addition to electrolytes. Excretion of these substances is not in general relevant in predicting the response to fluid management in dysnatremic states.

To derive the formula for CeH_2O, one substitutes electrolyte clearance (approximated by the clearance of the sum of sodium, potassium, and accompanying anions) for Cosm. Thus, the Cosm term is replaced by $C(Na + K) \times 2$. Analogous to Cosm,

$$C(Na + K) \times 2 = [U(Na + K) \times 2] \times V/P(Na + K) \times 2$$
$$= U(Na + K) \times V/P(Na + K)$$

Therefore,

$$CeH_2O = V - [U(Na + K) \times V/P(Na + K)]$$
$$= V\{1 - [U(Na + K)/PNa]\}$$

Note the K is dropped from the plasma term as it is numerically negligible.

Measurement of CeH_2O is very helpful in predicting the response to fluid therapy in dysnatremic states. This is particularly true in cases of hypernatremia (Leehey et al., 1989). This is best illustrated by some examples.

Take two patients with hypernatremia. They both have a plasma sodium concentration (PNa) of 160 mmol/L, a Posm of 350 mmol/kg, and a Uosm of 500 mmol/kg. Urine sodium concentration (UNa) and urine potassium concentration (UK) will vary depending on the situation. In *Patient 1*, the kidney is avidly reabsorbing sodium and water (UNa 10, UK 30; 24-hour urine volume 500 mL). This would be typical of a dehydrated hypotensive patient from a nursing home. In *Patient 2*, the kidney is excreting sodium and potassium and is polyuric (UNa 50, UK 30; 24-hour urine volume 4 L). This would be typical of an ICU patient who is recovering from shock who was previously resuscitated with many liters of saline and is now undergoing a solute diuresis (Bodonyi-Kovacs and Lecker, 2008; Sam et al., 2012).

In *Patient 1*:

$$CH_2O = V(1 - Uosm/Posm) = 0.5(1 - 500/350) = -0.21 \text{ L/day}$$

In *Patient 2*:

$$CH_2O = V(1 - Uosm/Posm) = 4(1 - 500/350) = -1.71 \text{ L/day}$$

In both cases, CH_2O is negative, that is, the kidney is reabsorbing free water. Negative free water clearance is the same as free water reabsorption and is termed TcH_2O. In fact, since V in the second patient is eightfold higher than that in the first patient, TcH_2O will also be eightfold higher.

Is the second patient really reabsorbing eight times as much water? Let us see what happens when CeH_2O is calculated:

In *Patient 1*:

$$CeH_2O = V\{1 - [U(Na + K)/PNa]\}$$
$$= 0.5[1 - (40/160)] = 0.375 \text{ L/day}$$

In *Patient 2*:

$$CeH_2O = V\{1 - [U(Na + K)/PNa]\} = 4[1 - (80/160)] = 2 \text{ L/day}$$

Now, we see that electrolyte-free water clearance is actually positive in both patients, that is, both are excreting electrolyte-free water in the urine; moreover, the second patient is excreting it almost six times as fast as the first patient. This is very important, since this indicates that both patients, but in particular the second patient, are actually losing water in the urine (not reabsorbing it!) and will have tendency to worsening hypernatremia unless they are given sufficient free water (Popli et al., 2014).

This discrepancy between CH_2O and CeH_2O is particularly marked in hypernatremic conditions—less so in hyponatremic ones.

Take two patients with hyponatremia. They both have a PNa of 120 mmol/L, a Posm of 250 mmol/kg, and a Uosm of 500 mmol/kg. In *Patient 1*, the kidney is avidly reabsorbing sodium and water (UNa 10, UK 30; 24-hour urine volume 500 mL/day). This would be typical of a hypotensive patient with gastrointestinal fluid losses. In *Patient 2*, there is a tumor-producing antidiuretic hormone (ADH), that is, the syndrome of inappropriate ADH (SIADH), and the kidney is excreting sodium and potassium but reabsorbing water (UNa 50, UK 50; 24-hour urine volume 1 L/day).

In *Patient 1*:

$$CH_2O = V(1 - Uosm/Posm) = 0.5(1 - 500/250)$$
$$= -0.5 \text{ L/day } (TcH_2O = 0.5 \text{ L/day})$$

In *Patient 2*:

$$CH_2O = V(1 - Uosm/Posm) = 1(1 - 500/250)$$
$$= -1.0 \text{ L/day } (TcH_2O = 1.0 \text{ L/day})$$

In both cases, CH_2O is negative, that is, TcH_2O is positive, and TcH_2O will be twofold higher in the second patient.

Let us see what happens when CeH_2O is calculated:
In *Patient 1*:

$$CeH_2O = V\{1 - [U(Na + K)/PNa]\} = 0.5[1 - (40/160)]$$
$$= 0.375 \text{ L/day}$$

Thus, this patient is actually appropriately excreting electrolyte-free water but not enough to correct the hyponatremia.
In *Patient 2*:

$$CeH_2O = V\{1 - [U(Na + K)/PNa]\}$$
$$= 1(1 - (80/160)) = 0.5 \text{ L/day}$$

Thus, even in the setting of SIADH, the kidney is excreting electrolyte-free water, but not enough to balance water intake.
Now let us see what might happen if physiologic saline is administered to these patients.

In *Patient 1*, the stimulus for ADH release (hypotension, hypovolemia) will be abrogated by the saline and the kidney will start to excrete electrolytes and water again. A typical response might be UNa 40, UK 25, Uosm 270, urine volume 2 L/day, and an improvement of PNa to 130 (Posm 270). Now,

$$CH_2O = V(1 - Uosm/Posm) = 2(1 - 270/270) = 0 \text{ L/day}$$

$$CeH_2O = V\{1 - [U(Na + K)/PNa]\} = 2[1 - (65/130)] = 1.0 \text{ L/day}$$

It can be seen that CH_2O predicts neither water loss nor gain by the kidney, whereas CeH_2O will predict that the kidney is now losing water. Thus, one must be careful once the patient starts diuresing not to correct the PNa too quickly.

In *Patient 2*, however, ADH release is independent of hemodynamic stimuli. Now the saline will be promptly excreted into the urine, but water will continue to be retained. A typical response might be UNa 150, UK 50, Uosm 600, urine volume 2 L/day, and no improvement (or even worsening) of PNa and Posm. If PNa decreases to 115 and Posm to 240:

$$CH_2O = V(1 - Uosm/Posm) = 2(1 - 600/240)$$
$$= -3.0 \text{ L/day (TcH}_2O \text{ 3.0 L/day)}$$

$$CeH_2O = V\{1 - [U(Na + K)/PNa]\} = 2[1 - (200/115)]$$
$$= -1.48 \text{ L/day (TcH}_2O \text{ 1.48 L/day)}$$

It can be seen that both CH_2O and CeH_2O indicate that the kidney will continue to retain water. This is why hyponatremia typically actually worsens when saline is administered to a patient with SIADH.

References

Bodonyi-Kovacs G, Lecker SH. Electrolyte-free water clearance: a key to the diagnosis of hypernatremia in resolving acute renal failure. *Clin Exp Nephrol.* 2008;12(1):74–78.

Goldberg M. Hyponatremia. *Med Clin North Am.* 1981;65(2):251–269.

Leehey DJ, Daugirdas JT, Manahan FJ, et al. Prolonged hypernatremia associated with azotemia
and hyponatriuria. *Am J Med.* 1989;86(4):494–496.

Popli S, Tzamaloukas AH, Ing TS. Osmotic diuresis-induced hypernatremia: better explained by
solute-free water clearance or electrolyte-free water clearance? *Int Urol Nephrol.* 2014;46(1):
207–210.

Sam R, Hart P, Haghighat R, et al. Hypervolemic hypernatremia in patients recovering from acute
kidney injury in the intensive care unit. *Clin Exp Nephrol.* 2012;16(1):136–146.

Smith HW. Renal excretion of sodium and water. *Fed Proc.* 1952;11(3):701–705.

9

How Does One Interpret the Urine Anion Gap and Urine Osmolal Gap?

The serum anion gap (AG) is a time-honored tool in nephrology. As discussed in Chapter 6, the AG is the difference between the plasma concentration of sodium, the major extracellular cation, and the sum of the concentrations of the major extracellular anions chloride and bicarbonate, that is, $[Na^+] - ([Cl^-] + [HCO_3^-])$. Stated differently, the *AG* occurs due to a higher concentration of unmeasured anions (i.e., not chloride or bicarbonate) than unmeasured cations (i.e., not sodium). The normal AG is about 10 to 14 mEq/L (see Fig. 6.1). Note that AG is usually expressed as milliequivalents per liter because it is a difference in charge.

The *urine AG* (UAG) is the difference between measured cations and anions in the urine (or the flip side, unmeasured anions and cations). However, as opposed to plasma, urine contains high concentrations of potassium and generally very small amounts of bicarbonate. Therefore, the UAG is $([Na^+] + [K^+]) - [Cl^-]$.

How is this helpful? It was initially postulated by Halperin and colleagues (Goldstein et al., 1986) that the UAG is a rough indicator of the amount of ammonium ion (NH_4^+) excreted in the urine. This is because in the absence of bicarbonate or another anion, NH_4^+ must be excreted with Cl^-. Thus, as urinary NH_4^+ increases, so will urinary Cl^-. Therefore, the lower (or more negative) the UAG, the more ammonium is in the urine.

A bit of renal physiology must be reviewed. Bicarbonate is freely filtered by the glomerulus and then almost completely reabsorbed (reclaimed) by the proximal tubule. Normally, there is little or no bicarbonate in the urine. So far, this seems like a "wash," that is, no gain or loss of bicarbonate. However, most of us eat what is called an "acid-ash" diet, which generates "nonvolatile" acid, which must be excreted by the kidneys. Such diets consist largely of meat or fish, eggs, and cereals with a lesser quantity of milk, fruit, and vegetables. Animal product consumption produces acid when catabolized due to the formation of sulfuric acid from an abundance of sulfur-containing amino acids (cysteine, cystine, and methionine) in animal proteins.

The role of the diet and its influence on the acidity of urine have been studied for decades. The French biologist Claude Bernard made the classical observation that changing the diet of rabbits from an herbivore to a carnivore diet changed the urine from more alkaline to more acid. Subsequent investigations focused on the chemical properties and acidity of constituents of the remains of foods combusted in a bomb calorimeter, described as ash. The "dietary ash hypothesis" proposed that foods, when metabolized, would leave a similar "acid ash" or "alkaline ash" in the body as those formed when the foods were oxidized in combustion (Dwyer et al., 1985).

It is generally stated that about 1 mEq/kg (mmol/kg) of "nonvolatile" acid is formed per day due to metabolism. This acid will consume an equal amount of body bicarbonate; this bicarbonate then must be regenerated by the distal nephron via renal acid excretion by one of the following three mechanisms:

1. Excretion of free H^+, thus lowering urine pH. This is minor mechanism; as even with a maximally acidic urine, the pH is only about 4.5, a $[H^+]$ of less than 0.04 mEq/L.
2. Excretion of H^+ in conjunction with an anion. This is predominantly phosphate via the reaction:

$$HPO_4^{2-} + H^+ \rightarrow H_2PO_4^-$$

3. Excretion of H^+ in conjunction with ammonia (NH_3). The main adaptive renal response to metabolic acidosis is to increase H^+ excretion in the form of NH_4^+. In patients with severe metabolic acidosis and normal renal function, NH_4^+ excretion can increase from the normal value of 30 to 40 mmol/day to as much as 200 to 300 mmol/day (Clarke et al., 1955).

Ammonium is usually excreted with chloride but is sometimes excreted with other anions such as ketoacid anions, hippurate, or bicarbonate. Since measurement of urinary NH_4^+ is not available in most clinical laboratories, the urinary $[NH_4^+]$ is generally estimated by its effects on the excretion of its accompanying anion (generally Cl^-). This led to the concept of the UAG, since there is a linear relationship between the UAG and urine $[NH_4^+]$. In response to an acid load, the UAG is normally -20 to -50 mEq/L in healthy subjects. Later, the terminology *urine net charge* instead of *UAG* was used, with the normal response to acidosis being a negative *net charge*.

Metabolic acidosis of renal origin in the absence of renal failure, called renal tubular acidosis (RTA), can result from the failure of proximal bicarbonate reabsorption or distal acid excretion (Table 9.1).

- Hypokalemic distal RTA (type 1) is due to impaired secretion of H^+ from the alpha-intercalated cells in the collecting duct, thus impairing distal tubular bicarbonate regeneration. Increased secretion of K^+ also occurs, resulting in hypokalemic hyperchloremic acidosis. The most common causes are hereditary, autoimmune disease, tubulointerstitial disease, and dysproteinemias. Other findings include increased urine pH (>5.3) despite systemic acidosis; decreased NH_4^+ excretion, resulting in decreased excretion of the accompanying chloride anion; and thus urinary $([Na^+] + [K^+]) > [Cl^-]$ (positive UAG or "net charge").
- Proximal RTA (type 2) is due to failure to reabsorb filtered bicarbonate. It is often accompanied by other evidence of proximal tubule dysfunction, or Fanconi syndrome (hypouricemia, hypophosphatemia, renal glycosuria). The most common causes are dysproteinemias and drugs that block carbonic anhydrase, an enzyme which facilitates proximal bicarbonate reabsorption (carbonic anhydrase inhibitors). Other findings include urine pH <5.3; UAG ("net charge") is variable and cannot be used for diagnosis. Urine pH is generally acidic since previous loss of bicarbonate into the urine has lowered plasma bicarbonate and the resulting decreased filtered load of bicarbonate can now be reabsorbed by the proximal tubule.

TABLE 9.1   Characteristic Laboratory Findings in Renal Tubular Acidosis

	Renal Tubular Acidosis		
	Type 1	Type 2	Type 4
Plasma K^+	Low	Low	High
Urine pH	>5.3	<5.3	<5.3
Urine anion gap (net charge)	Positive	Variable	Positive
Plasma aldosterone/K^+ ratio	Normal	Normal	Usually low (unless aldosterone resistance)

- Hyperkalemic distal RTA (type 4) is usually due to hypoaldosteronism or aldosterone resistance in the setting of chronic kidney disease (CKD). The resultant hyperkalemia leads to decreased NH_4^+ excretion (due to inhibition of ammonia formation). The most common causes are diabetes (hyporeninemic hypoaldosteronism due to glycation of prorenin with impaired activation to renin) and drugs, including renin–angiotensin system (RAS) blockers, aldosterone synthesis inhibitors such as heparin, and inhibitors of tubular K^+ secretion such as trimethoprim and calcineurin inhibitors. Nonsteroidal anti-inflammatory drugs (NSAIDs) inhibit the RAS as well as tubular K^+ secretion. Other findings include urine pH <5.3; and urinary $([Na^+] + [K^+]) >$ $[Cl^-]$ (positive UAG or "net charge"). A diagnosis of hypoaldosteronism needs to be confirmed by measurement of plasma aldosterone levels.

The utility of the UAG in the diagnosis of hyperchloremic (non-AG) metabolic acidosis is illustrated in the cases that follow.

PATIENT 1

A 60-year-old man presents with metabolic acidosis. He gives a history of diarrhea. His laboratory values reveal (in mmol/L) Na^+ 140, K^+ 2.5, Cl^- 120, and total CO_2 10. The urine pH is 6.

Q: What is the expected UAG (urine "net charge")?

A: In general, urinary $([Na^+] + [K^+]) > [Cl^-]$ in healthy individuals, generally by 20 to 90 mmol/L. If one has metabolic acidosis due to diarrhea, the normal renal response will be to increase NH_3 production and NH_4^+ excretion. Thus, we expect $([Na^+] + [K^+]) < [Cl^-]$ and a low urine pH. However, if the distal tubule is the problem, then $([Na^+] + [K^+]) > [Cl^-]$, and the urine pH will be >5.3 despite metabolic acidosis.

In some cases of diarrhea-induced hyperchloremic metabolic acidosis, however, especially when hypokalemia also develops, the urine pH may be high (>5.3), erroneously suggesting the presence of a RTA. This occurs because of impaired distal delivery of sodium (due to volume depletion), which leads to less H^+ excretion into the urine. Correction of the volume deficit results in acidification of the urine in such patients with the fall in urine pH associated with an increase in the urinary sodium concentration. For instance, if urinary $[Na^+]$ is <25 mmol/L, urinary pH is >5.3, but urine pH decreases to <5.3 when urine $[Na^+]$ is increased to >25 mmol/L. Thus, in this setting, a negative UAG correctly points to diarrhea rather than impaired urinary acidification (RTA) as the etiology of the metabolic acidosis (Batlle et al., 1988).

In some situations, anions other than chloride may be excreted with ammonium. In these cases, UAG can be misleading, and *urine osmolal gap* (UOG) may be needed to assess urinary ammonium excretion. Examples of these unmeasured anions are ketoacid anions (beta-hydroxybutyrate and acetoacetate), bicarbonate (when proximal RTA is treated with alkali therapy), or hippurate (from glue-sniffing and subsequent toluene metabolism). Theoretically, excretion of L-lactate anions (in the setting of lactic acidosis) would also limit chloride excretion, which could suggest the presence of an RTA when the real cause of acidosis is overproduction of lactic acid. Since L-lactate is avidly reabsorbed by renal tubules, this does not usually occur; however, D-lactic acidosis, a rare condition due to intestinal bacterial production of D-lactic acid in short bowel syndrome, will lead to excretion of D-lactate and can mimic RTA.

Thus, the UOG can be used to assess changes in ammonium excretion concentration regardless of the accompanying anion (Halperin and Kamel, 2010). The calculation of UOG compares the measured urine osmolality to an estimate of the urine osmolality calculated from the sum of the urine concentrations of sodium, potassium, urea nitrogen (or urea), and, if the dipstick is glucose positive, glucose, using the following formula:

Calculated urine osmolality (mmol/L)
  = $(2 \times [Na^+ + K^+])$ + [Urine urea nitrogen in mg/dL]/2.8
    + [Urine glucose in mg/dL]/18

Or, more simply, if standard international units (mmol/L) are used:

Calculated urine osmolality (mmol/L) = $(2 \times [Na^+ + K^+])$
                                       + [Urea] + [Glucose]

UOG = Measured urine osmolality − Calculated urine osmolality

Ammonium makes up about 50% of the UOG (some prefer the term "modified UOG" that is UOG/2). The normal value of the UOG is 10 to 100 mmol/L; urine $[NH_4^+]$ should be approximately one-half this value, that is, 5 to 50 mmol/L. Ammonium excretion and thus UOG should markedly increase with metabolic acidosis of nonrenal etiology. A UOG <150 mmol/L in a patient with metabolic acidosis suggests impairment of ammonium excretion, as with a distal RTA. A UOG >400 mmol/L (urine $[NH_4^+]$ >200 mmol/L) is typical of diarrhea-induced metabolic acidosis (in the absence of renal disease).

PATIENT 2

A 30-year-old woman is brought to the ER by her boyfriend because of altered mental status. Her laboratory values reveal (in mmol/L) Na^+ 140, K^+ 2.5, Cl^- 120, and total CO_2 10. The urine pH is 6. The UAG is +50 mmol/L and UOG is +300 mmol/L.

Q: What is your diagnosis?

A: The metabolic acidosis generated by toluene inhalation (such as glue-sniffing) is a good example of a condition in which the UOG is necessary to arrive at the correct diagnosis. Toluene is metabolized primarily to hippuric acid. Retention of the acid anion hippurate might be expected to result in a high AG metabolic acidosis (similar to the situation with lactic acidosis and ketoacidosis). However, with normal or near-normal renal function, hippurate is rapidly excreted in the urine by both glomerular filtration and tubular secretion. Initially, hippurate is excreted with sodium and potassium; in this phase, the UOG will be normal and the UAG will be positive (i.e., $([Na^+] + [K^+]) > [Cl^-]$). With time, due to metabolic acidosis, ammonium excretion progressively increases and, in large part, is excreted as ammonium hippurate (rather than ammonium chloride). The UAG will remain positive in this setting, erroneously suggesting impairment in ammonium excretion and the presence of a RTA. However, the UOG will progressively increase due to excretion of ammonium with hippurate. In addition, increased potassium excretion with hippurate may lead to hypokalemia and a further increase in renal ammoniagenesis. As a result, there will be more NH_3 to bind with H^+ to form NH_4^+, and the urine pH can increase to >5.5 or higher. In this situation, the combination of hyperchloremic acidosis, positive UAG, and high urine pH suggests distal RTA, and only the large UOG will point to the correct diagnosis of overproduction of hippuric acid due to toluene abuse.

There are known difficulties with estimation of urine ammonium excretion by UOG. For instance, there may be other osmotically-active substances besides ammonium in the urine (e.g., alcohols) that can increase the UOG. If the urine is infected by a urea-splitting organism, NH_4^+ formed by the bacteria can increase the UOG as well as the pH. Moreover, calculation of the UOG is not able to detect small changes in urine ammonium excretion.

In view of all of these difficulties, why not just directly measure urinary $[NH_4^+]$? In these days of automation, many clinical laboratories do not offer this test. However, it is possible to predilute the urine by 1:100 or greater, thereby enabling measurement of urine $[NH_4^+]$ using an autoanalyzer (Kraut and Madias, 2012). This should probably be done more often in clinical laboratories.

References

Batlle DC, Hizon M, Cohen E, et al. The use of the urinary anion gap in the diagnosis of hyperchloremic metabolic acidosis. *N Engl J Med*. 1988;318(10):594–599.

Clarke E, Evans BM, Macintyre I, et al. Acidosis in experimental electrolyte depletion. *Clin Sci (Lond)*. 1955;14(3):421–440.

Dwyer J, Foulkes E, Evans M, et al. Acid/alkaline ash diets: time for assessment and change. *J Am Diet Assoc*. 1985;85(7):841–845.

Goldstein MB, Bear R, Richardson RM, et al. The urine anion gap: a clinically useful index of ammonium excretion. *Am J Med Sci*. 1986;292(4):198–202.

Halperin ML, Kamel KS. Some observations on the clinical approach to metabolic acidosis. *J Am Soc Nephrol*. 2010;21:894–897.

Kraut JA, Madias NE. Differential diagnosis of nongap metabolic acidosis: value of a systematic approach. *Clin J Am Soc Nephrol*. 2012;7(4):671–679.

Is It "Acute Renal Failure" or "Acute Kidney Injury"?

10

For decades, nephrologists used the term *acute renal failure (ARF)*, defined as a sudden (within hours to days) decrease in renal function, leading to retention of nitrogenous waste products (e.g., urea and creatinine). Classically, ARF was divided into prerenal failure (decreased renal blood flow leading to decreased glomerular filtration rate), postrenal failure (urinary obstruction), and intrinsic renal failure, due to injury to kidney tissue, most commonly tubules (acute tubular necrosis [ATN]) but also interstitial cells (acute interstitial nephritis [AIN]), and less commonly glomeruli (acute glomerulonephritis), or blood vessels (acute vasculopathy/vasculitis).

More recently, the term *acute kidney injury (AKI)* has been used instead of *ARF* or *ATN*. However, since not all patients with ARF have kidney injury, and there are no biochemical markers of kidney injury in widespread clinical use in the United States at this time, the term *AKI* as currently used is a bit of a misnomer.

Several consensus definitions of AKI have been developed in an attempt to provide a uniform definition. In 2004, the Acute Dialysis Quality Initiative (ADQI) group, which included expert intensivists as well as nephrologists, proposed a consensus graded definition, called the RIFLE criteria (Bellomo et al., 2004). A modification of the RIFLE criteria was subsequently proposed by the Acute Kidney Injury Network (AKIN) (Mehta et al., 2007). More recently, the Kidney Disease: Improving Global Outcomes (KDIGO) AKI Workgroup also proposed a definition (KDIGO, 2012) (Table 10.1).

According to AKIN diagnostic criteria for AKI, an increase in the serum creatinine concentration of as little as 0.3 mg/dL (26.4 μmol/L)

	Creatinine (RIFLE)	Creatinine (AKIN)	Creatinine (KDIGO)	Urine Output
Definition	>50% increase within 7 d	>50% increase *or* increase of 0.3 mg/dL within 48 h	>50% increase within 7 d *or* increase of 0.3 mg/dL within 48 h	<0.5 mL/kg/h for >6 h
Staging				
AKIN/KDIGO Stage 1; RIFLE-Risk	>50% increase	>50% increase *or* increase of 0.3 mg/dL	>50% increase *or* increase of 0.3 mg/dL	<0.5 mL/kg/h for >6 h
AKIN/KDIGO Stage 2; RIFLE-Injury	>100% increase	>100% increase	>100% increase	<0.5 mL/kg/h for >12 h
AKIN/KDIGO Stage 3; RIFLE-Failure	>200% increase	>200% increase	>200% increase	<0.3 mL/kg/h for >12 h *or* anuria for >12 h
RIFLE-Loss	Need for dialysis for >4 wk			
RIFLE-End-stage	Need for dialysis for >3 mo			

from baseline, or a 1.5-fold or greater increase in serum creatinine over 48 hours, or oliguria (<0.5 mL/kg/h) for more than 6 hours is sufficient to establish the diagnosis. However, these criteria should be applied only after volume status had been optimized and urinary tract obstruction excluded. KDIGO added the modification that the 1.5-fold increase in serum creatinine could develop over less than 7 days instead of less than 48 hours. According to KDIGO, AKI can include various etiologies of acute renal dysfunction, including prerenal azotemia, ATN, AIN, acute glomerular and vasculitic renal diseases, and acute postrenal obstructive nephropathy. The inclusion of very small increments in serum creatinine in the diagnostic criteria was based on epidemiologic data, showing that such patients have worse outcomes (Newsome et al., 2008)

There have been many concerns regarding the use of these criteria to diagnose AKI. In particular, brief durations of oliguria may be due to insufficient fluid administration and not kidney injury. Another concern is the difficulty in calculation of change in serum creatinine in patients who present with AKI without a baseline measurement of serum creatinine. However, the most important concern is the use of functional markers, that is, serum creatinine and urine output, to define injury. The aforementioned definitions are likely leading to an increase in the number of nephrology consultations for AKI and an increase in reported incidence of AKI in hospitalized patients that may not be clinically important (Palevsky et al., 2013). Very small changes in serum creatinine may reflect hemodynamic changes, fluid shifts, or even laboratory variability rather than clinically important disease.

There is also an inherent problem in assigning patients into various stages of AKI based on serum creatinine changes from baseline. This is because serum creatinine will continue to increase, usually for 48 to 72 hours, after GFR is already starting to improve (see Fig. 2.2). Thus, it might appear that the stage of AKI is worsening when in reality renal function is improving.

So, what is the answer to the question: is it ARF or AKI? The author believes that the term *AKI* should be used to describe the condition formerly called *intrinsic ARF* (the term *ATN* is outmoded, as it implies a pathologic change that may or may not be present). Another term that would logically apply to conditions resulting in a sudden (within hours to days) decrease in renal function would be *acute kidney disease*, although this term is not in widespread use. The nephrology community still awaits the "renal troponin" or "renal troponins" that will hopefully definitively determine if renal injury has indeed occurred. In this regard, it is of interest that KDIGO now uses the acronym *AKI* to mean either *acute kidney injury* or *acute kidney impairment*.

PATIENT 1

A 65-year-old man undergoes three-vessel coronary artery bypass grafting. His serum creatinine is 1 mg/dL preoperatively. He does well postoperatively, but on the second day post-op his serum creatinine is noted to be 1.3 mg/dL. Urinalysis is normal except for moderate hyaline casts, and fractional excretion of urea (FEurea) is 20%. Urine output is 2 L daily, and he has no edema. Diuretics are stopped, and within 2 days the serum creatinine is again 1 mg/dL. He recovers from surgery uneventfully and is discharged on the fourth hospital day.

Q: Does this patient have *AKI*?

A: According to the AKIN and KDIGO criteria, the answer is yes, as the serum creatinine increased by 0.3 mg/dL within 48 hours. However, there is no evidence of renal injury on urinalysis, and the history of diuretic use, low FEurea, and rapid improvement of renal function with diuretic cessation points to a prerenal etiology. The AKIN criteria are that prerenal failure should be excluded before making the diagnosis of AKI, whereas KDIGO now has broadened the definition of *AKI* to encompass *acute kidney impairment* as well as *acute kidney injury* (convenient!). The important thing from a clinical standpoint is that the patient recovered quickly and went home at his baseline serum creatinine. Most clinicians would not call this a disease, and not label it AKI.

PATIENT 2

A 75-year-old woman is hospitalized for an acute systemic illness consisting of low-grade fever, arthralgias, skin rash, and dyspnea. On examination, she has bilateral chest rales and lower extremity petechiae. Urinalysis reveals proteinuria, hematuria, and granular casts. Her serum creatinine is 3 mg/dL and was 1.5 mg/dL 1 week previously.

Q: Does this patient have *AKI*?

A: This patient makes KDIGO criteria for AKI due to more than 50% increase in serum creatinine within 7 days. Definitions aside, what is important to realize here is that there is clearly kidney injury as manifested by urinalysis findings coupled with rising serum creatinine. On clinical grounds, either acute glomerulonephritis or vasculitis was suspected. A test for antineutrophil cytoplasmic antibodies (ANCAs) was positive, and renal biopsy revealed pauci-immune necrotizing crescentic vasculitis. She was treated with high-dose steroids and cyclophosphamide with recovery of renal function.

References

Bellomo R, Ronco C, Kellum JA, et al. Acute renal failure—definition, outcome measures, animal models, fluid therapy and information technology needs: the Second International Consensus Conference of the Acute Dialysis Quality Initiative (ADQI) Group. *Crit Care.* 2004;8:R204.

KDIGO. KDIGO clinical practice guideline for acute kidney injury. *Kidney Int Suppl.* 2012;2:8.

Mehta RL, Kellum JA, Shah SV, et al. Acute Kidney Injury Network: report of an initiative to improve outcomes in acute kidney injury. *Crit Care.* 2007;11:R31.

Newsome BB, Warnock DG, McClellan WM, et al. Longterm risk of mortality and end-stage renal disease among the elderly after small increases in serum creatinine level during hospitalization for acute myocardial infarction. *Arch Intern Med.* 2008;168(6):609–616.

Palevsky PM, Liu KD, Brophy PD, et al. KDOQI US commentary on the 2012 KDIGO clinical practice guideline for acute kidney injury. *Am J Kidney Dis.* 2013;61:649–672.

11

What Exactly Is Dialysis and When Is It Needed?

A frequent reason for inpatient nephrology consultation is either a need for dialysis (in a patient with end-stage renal disease [ESRD] who is hospitalized) or a wish for the nephrologist to consider dialysis (for instance, in a patient with severe chronic kidney disease [CKD] or acute kidney injury [AKI]).

First, let us consider what the term *dialysis* means. The word comes from a combination of the Greek words *dia* and *lysis*, which translate into English as *through* and *splitting*, respectively. The word *dialysis* thus reflects the fact that the procedure involves "splitting" of solutes from blood passing across a semipermeable membrane, the solute diffusing "through" the membrane along its concentration gradient. Diffusion is bidirectional, meaning that a given solute can be either removed or added to the blood. Most of the time, a solute is being removed since its concentration in uremic blood is higher than the concentration in the fluid placed on the other side of the membrane, which is termed dialysate. Examples of such solutes are urea, creatinine, and (usually) potassium. However, in other instances, the solute concentration in dialysate is generally higher than that in the blood, such as with bicarbonate and (often) calcium. Removal of fluid is not achieved by dialysis, but rather by *ultrafiltration*, which means removal of an ultrafiltrate of plasma (i.e., plasma water containing smaller molecular weight solutes, but not larger molecular weight solutes and proteins). Dialysis results in changes in the plasma concentrations of the solutes either removed or added to the plasma. On the other hand, with ultrafiltration using hemodialysis equipment, a hydrostatic pressure gradient is employed to induce the filtration (or convection) of plasma water across the membrane of the hemofilter. The frictional force between water and solutes (called solvent drag) results in the convective transport of small- and middle-molecular-weight solutes across the membrane along with the water. An important difference between convection and diffusion is that with convection, solute removal is determined by the pore size of the membrane, whereas with diffusion, efficiency of solute removal is greatest with smaller molecules at any given pore size. When ultrafiltration is performed without dialysis, this is termed isolated ultrafiltration (IUF). With IUF, solutes are present in the ultrafiltrate at the same or similar concentrations to those of the plasma and, as opposed to dialysis, plasma concentration of these solutes will not change due to the procedure.

Many patients and some clinicians are uncertain of the distinction between dialysis and ultrafiltration. Indeed, nephrologists are often requested to "dialyze" patients, when in fact what is desired is fluid removal. Possibly the term "blood purification" (English translation of Chinese term for dialysis) or even "blood cleaning" (pure English!) would be preferable to continuing to speak in Greek. At least this would make clear to patients and practitioners what "dialysis" is really doing.

There are two forms of dialysis: hemodialysis and peritoneal dialysis. Both are effective and widely used for maintenance dialysis, though hemodialysis results in faster solute removal and more predictable fluid removal and is preferred in most acute settings.

WHAT ARE THE INDICATIONS FOR DIALYSIS?

Maintenance Dialysis

The decision to start maintenance dialysis is based upon the presence of ESRD-related signs and symptoms, the estimated glomerular filtration rate (eGFR), the rate of decline of the eGFR, and clinical judgment. Symptoms and signs attributable to kidney failure include serositis (such as pericarditis and pleuritis), acid–base or electrolyte disorders not easily corrected by medical management, dysgeusia (altered taste), severe pruritus, hiccoughs, refractory volume overload, progressive deterioration in nutritional status, or cognitive impairment. In the past, asymptomatic patients with eGFR less than $10 \text{ mL}/\text{min}/1.73 \text{ m}^2$ were often started on maintenance dialysis even in the absence of symptoms or signs of uremia or fluid overload. This practice has changed somewhat as the result of findings of the Initiating Dialysis Early and Late (IDEAL) study, a randomized clinical trial in which planned early initiation of dialysis in patients with stage 5 CKD was not associated with an improvement in survival or clinical outcomes (Cooper et al., 2010). In this study, 828 patients with an eGFR between 10 and $15 \text{ mL}/\text{min}/1.73 \text{ m}^2$

were randomly assigned to dialysis initiation when the eGFR was either 10 to 14 mL/min/1.73 m^2 or 5 to 7 mL/min/1.73 m^2. Dialysis was initiated on the basis of the presence of uremic symptoms and volume overload as well as on the eGFR. Since the majority of patients assigned to the late-start arm initiated dialysis when the eGFR was greater than 5 to 7 mL/min/1.73 m^2, the mean eGFR was 9.8 mL/min/1.73 m^2 at the start of dialysis for the late-start group versus 12 mL/min/1.73 m^2 in the early-start arm. On the basis of this study, most nephrologists do not initiate maintenance dialysis in the absence of signs or symptoms of uremia or fluid overload. However, if the eGFR is very low ($\leq$5 mL/min/1.73 m^2), many nephrologists will start maintenance dialysis even in the absence of symptoms due to risk of complications in seemingly asymptomatic patients. Absolute indications to start dialysis include uremic pericarditis or pleuritis or uremic encephalopathy.

Since eGFR is determined on the basis of population studies, in selected patients, a 24-hour urine for measurement of urea and creatinine clearance may be performed in order to provide a more accurate estimate of the GFR. In the absence of congestive heart failure, the mean of the urea and creatinine clearance is very similar to the GFR measured by inulin clearance in patients with severe CKD (GFR < 20 mL/min) (Lubowitz et al., 1967). In some centers, GFR can be determined by clearance of an exogenous substance that is excreted by glomerular filtration and neither reabsorbed nor secreted by renal tubules (e.g., inulin, iohexol, iothalamate, diethylene triamine pentaacetic acid).

Acute Dialysis

The decision to perform dialysis on a patient with acute renal failure or acute worsening of CKD is based on clinical judgment, as there are no randomized trials for guidance. As opposed to maintenance dialysis, eGFR plays little or no role in the decision process. There is a helpful mnemonic used on rounds—AEIOU.

A—**A**cidosis (occasionally severe alkalosis)

Dialysis fluid (dialysate) used for hemodialysis contains bicarbonate, usually at a concentration of about 35 mmol/L. Therefore, hemodialysis is very effective at correcting metabolic acidosis. Most dialysis machines can adjust the bicarbonate concentration down to about 28 to 30 mmol/L and up to about 40 mmol/L. Use of the lower bicarbonate concentration can be used to correct severe metabolic alkalosis. Peritoneal dialysate contains lactate, which must be metabolized to produce bicarbonate in the body.

E—**E**lectrolyte disturbance

The most important electrolyte disturbance for which dialysis is performed is hyperkalemia, as severe hyperkalemia can lead to electrocardiographic changes and cardiac arrest. The advisability of rapid correction of hyperkalemia requires clinical judgment and is discussed in Chapter 15. Other electrolyte disturbances occasionally necessitating urgent dialysis are severe hypercalcemia, hyperphosphatemia, and hypermagnesemia. More rapid correction is achieved by hemodialysis than by peritoneal dialysis.

I—**I**ntoxications (when the intoxicant is dialyzable, and enough will be removed to affect patient outcome)

Hemodialysis should be used rather than peritoneal dialysis for intoxications as higher clearance rates can be achieved. In general, dialysis is best used to remove small-molecular-weight toxins that are not bound to plasma proteins (therefore, readily dialyzable) and that have a relatively small volume of distribution (so that a meaningful amount of the total body burden of toxin can be removed). Also, some toxins (such as methanol) exert their most serious toxicity once they are metabolized to other substances (in this case, formic acid and formaldehyde); dialytic removal of the parent compound will prevent conversion to these toxic metabolites. Examples of substances for which dialysis is of clinical benefit for treatment of intoxications are lithium, methanol, ethylene glycol, and salicylate.

O—Fluid **O**verload (this is actually an indication for ultrafiltration)

Both hemodialysis and peritoneal dialysis are effective means of fluid removal, though the amount of fluid removed is more predictable with hemodialysis as the desired ultrafiltration rate can be dialed into the machine. With peritoneal dialysis, fluid removal is achieved by maintaining an osmotic gradient between the dialysate and blood (generally by using high concentrations of dextrose in the dialysate), and the amount of fluid removed will be affected by the peritoneal membrane transport characteristics of the particular patient being treated.

In practice, both dialysis and ultrafiltration are usually carried out in tandem during hemodialysis. However, it is possible to perform isovolumic hemodialysis (i.e., without fluid removal) as well as IUF using hemodialysis equipment.

U—**U**remia

As discussed earlier, uremia is a clinical syndrome, encompassing a protean array of symptoms and signs, including anorexia, dysgeusia hiccoughs, pruritus, nausea and vomiting, pericarditis, bleeding, and cognitive/neurologic impairment. Uremic manifestations are thought to be primarily due to accumulation of waste products of protein metabolism, though it is not known which substance(s) actually lead to uremia. Urea and creatinine are minimally toxic and nontoxic, respectively, and plasma levels correlate only roughly with uremic manifestations. An elevation in plasma urea nitrogen and creatinine is termed azotemia, whereas uremia necessitates the presence of symptoms and/or signs and is a clinical diagnosis. When dialyzing patients with uremic symptoms and signs, one must take care not to lower the plasma urea nitrogen levels too quickly, as rapid removal of osmotically active particles from the plasma can lead to movement of water into cells and brain swelling, resulting in headache, seizures, and even death.

The case studies that follow will point out some of the more quantitative aspects of dialysis.

CHRONIC HEMODIALYSIS

PATIENT 1

A 70-kg male patient with ESRD has a plasma urea nitrogen concentration (usually called blood urea nitrogen or "BUN" in the United States) of 100 mg/dL. The clinician wishes to lower the concentration of urea and other solutes but remove no net fluid.

Urea is a low-molecular-weight solute and a product of protein metabolism. Although it not particularly toxic, there is a rough correlation between the level of urea in the blood and the presence of uremic symptoms. Urea kinetic methodology is therefore utilized to assess adequacy of dialysis.

The molecular weight of urea is 60 Da, and the molecular structure is as follows:

$$\underset{H_2N}{\overset{\displaystyle \overset{O}{\|}}{}} \underset{\qquad}{\overset{C}{}} NH_2$$

It can be seen that there are two nitrogen (N) atoms in each molecule of urea. Since the atomic weight of N is 14, the atomic weight of the urea nitrogens in urea is 28. In other countries, urea rather than urea nitrogen is usually measured. A plasma urea nitrogen of 100 mg/dL equals 214 mg/dL (36 mmol/L) of urea.

Since urea distributes into the total body water (0.6 × body weight in kg, or 42 L in this patient), the body content of urea nitrogen at the beginning of dialysis in this patient is 1,000 mg/L × 42 L = 42 g.

First let us assume that the patient's blood was completely cleaned (i.e., all the urea was removed) on one pass through the dialyzer. In this instance, removal of 21 g of urea nitrogen would lower the concentration of plasma urea nitrogen to 50 mg/dL and removal of all 42 g of urea nitrogen would lower the plasma urea nitrogen to 0. This does not really happen, as there is a hemodialysis circuit whereby blood is recirculated again and again through the dialyzer, thus lowering the efficiency of the blood cleaning. It turns out that running 42 L of plasma through the dialyzer will lead to only a 63% reduction of plasma urea nitrogen. In dialysis parlance, we would say that urea clearance/volume of distribution of urea or Kt/V (where Kt = urea clearance and V = volume of distribution of urea) in this patient is 42 L/42 L = 1, which will result in a urea reduction ratio (URR) of 63%. Thus, 42 g $\times$ 0.63 = 26.5 g of urea nitrogen will be removed. It should be noted that other factors will affect Kt/V, such as urea generation and ultrafiltration rate during dialysis and the amount of urea rebound after dialysis (due to shift of urea from cells and interstitial fluid into the blood), but we will not be concerned with these issues here.

Now let us consider the effect of IUF on urea clearance in Patient 2.

PATIENT 2

A 70-kg male postoperative patient was given 20 L of fluid in the operating room and is in pulmonary edema. He is oliguric. The plasma urea nitrogen is 20 mg/dL. The clinician wishes to remove fluid but does not need to clean the blood. The nephrologist orders IUF, with 4 L of fluid to be removed during 4 hours (1 L/h). How much urea nitrogen is being removed?

In this case, an ultrafiltrate of plasma (plasma water, electrolytes, and other small-molecular-weight substances such as urea that can pass through the pores of the dialyzer membrane) will be removed, but there is no diffusion of solute across the dialyzer membrane. The concentration of urea nitrogen in the ultrafiltrate is not usually measured, but will generally be very similar to the concentration in the plasma. In this patient, the amount of urea nitrogen removed will only be 200 mg/L $\times$ 4 L = 800 mg, and there will be no change in plasma urea nitrogen.

Now let us return to Patient 1. If the nephrologist had also ordered 4 L of fluid to be removed during hemodialysis, the total amount of urea nitrogen removed would be the 26.5 g removed by diffusion plus the amount of urea nitrogen removed in the ultrafiltrate by convection. The actual amount removed during "dialytic ultrafiltration" will vary depending on factors such as blood flow rate and dialysate flow rate, and the concentration of urea nitrogen will be somewhat lower in the ultrafiltrate than in the plasma. Assuming the average plasma urea nitrogen during the dialysis is 75 mg/dL, one can see that the maximum amount of urea nitrogen in the ultrafiltrate would be about 750 mg/L $\times$ 4 L or about 3 g. Thus, ultrafiltration has a relatively small effect on total urea nitrogen removal during the hemodialysis procedure. Therefore, if it is necessary to clean the blood in fluid-overloaded patients, one must perform simultaneous dialysis and ultrafiltration ("dialytic ultafiltration"), not just ultrafiltration.

CHRONIC PERITONEAL DIALYSIS

With peritoneal dialysis, the dialyzer is not an artificial filter but the peritoneal membrane. Peritoneal dialysis is performed by placing dialysate into the peritoneal cavity, after which toxins from the splanchnic circulation are allowed to diffuse across the peritoneal membrane into the dialysate, which is then discarded. As mentioned earlier, the mechanism of fluid removal is not a hydraulic pressure gradient but rather an osmotic pressure gradient across the membrane. The osmotic gradient is created by adding solute (usually dextrose) to the dialysate so that the osmolality of the dialysate is greater than that of the plasma, thus causing loss of water and accompanying solutes into the dialysate. Peritoneal dialysis thus involves simultaneous diffusion dialysis and osmotic ultrafiltration. As opposed to hemodialysis, with peritoneal dialysis, changes in ultrafiltration volume can have a clinically important effect on solute removal.

PATIENT 3

A 70-kg anuric male patient with ESRD on chronic ambulatory peritoneal dialysis (CAPD) has a plasma urea nitrogen of 50 mg/dL. He uses 2 L exchanges of 1.5% dextrose-containing dialysate (osmolality 346 mmol/kg) every 6 hours (i.e., 4 exchanges/day). His total daily dialysate volume is 8 L, that is, there is no net ultrafiltration. Assuming the dialysate concentration of urea nitrogen is also 50 mg/dL, what is the daily urea clearance? (The dialysate concentration is, in reality, slightly lower than the plasma concentration in most patients, but we will assume here that there was complete equilibration across the peritoneal membrane.)

Since with peritoneal dialysis, the spent dialysate contains urea at approximately the same concentration as that found in the plasma, the daily dialysate volume (in this case, 8 L) will be approximately the same as the daily urea clearance. Thus,

$$\text{Daily} \quad Kt/V = 8\,L/42\,L = 0.19, \text{ and}$$
$$\text{Weekly} \quad Kt/V = 0.19 \times 7 = 1.3$$

A number of studies have demonstrated that weekly Kt/V should be more than or equal to 1.7 in peritoneal dialysis patients; thus this patient does not have adequate dialytic urea clearance. But now let us assume that there is 2 L of net ultrafiltration daily. Now,

$$\text{Daily } Kt/V = 10\text{ L}/42\text{ L} = 0.24, \text{ or a weekly } Kt/V \text{ of } 1.7,$$
$$\text{which is adequate}$$

All patients in the United States with ESRD are maintained on either hemodialysis or peritoneal dialysis. In Europe, some ESRD patients are maintained on chronic hemofiltration. However, acute hemofiltration is commonly used in patients with AKI throughout the world, as will now be discussed.

ACUTE DIALYSIS

In the acute care setting in the ICU, standard intermittent hemodialysis (IHD) (generally for 4 hours) and peritoneal dialysis can still be performed, just as with ESRD outpatients. Some clinicians like to employ extended IHD (generally for 8–12 hours), often called sustained low-efficiency hemodialysis (SLED), in order to decrease the rate of solute and fluid removal. In severely ill patients with hemodynamic instability, many clinicians prefer to use continuous renal replacement therapy (CRRT). As the name would imply, CRRT is at least theoretically "continuous," that is, a "24/7" procedure. Various modifications of CRRT have been used, in which extended but not continuous (i.e., <24-hour) therapies are performed using CRRT equipment. For simplicity, we will stick with the classic CRRT therapies for the remainder of the discussion.

The CRRT modalities commonly used in the ICU are continuous venovenous hemodialysis (CVVHD) and continuous venovenous hemofiltration (CVVH). Since all CRRT techniques now utilize a double-lumen catheter placed in a large vein, some prefer to use the simpler terms continuous hemodialysis (C-HD) and continuous hemofiltration (C-HF). If the two procedures are combined, this is called continuous venovenous hemodiafiltration (CVVHDF) or more simply continuous hemodiafiltration (C-HDF). Analogous to IUF performed using standard hemodialysis equipment, one can perform continuous venovenous ultrafiltration (CVVU), more commonly called slow continuous ultrafiltration (SCUF), if only fluid removal is desired (Fig. 11.1).

What Is the Difference between Hemodialysis and Hemofiltration?
The answer is plenty, though they look similar at the bedside (Figs. 11.2 and 11.3). Whereas with CVVHD, dialysate (also called replacement

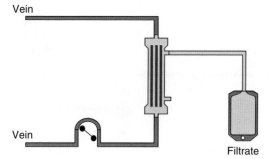

FIGURE 11.1 Slow continuous ultrafiltration. (Adapted from Bellomo R, Ronco C, Mehta RL. Nomenclature for continuous renal replacement therapies. *Am J Kidney Dis.* 1996;28(5):S2–S7.)

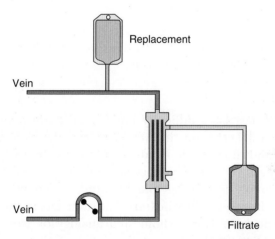

FIGURE 11.2 Continuous venovenous hemofiltration, with replacement fluid given "post-filter." (Adapted from Bellomo R, Ronco C, Mehta RL. Nomenclature for continuous renal replacement therapies. *Am J Kidney Dis.* 1996;28(5):S2–S7.)

fluid) is run through the dialyzer and solute is removed by diffusion (just like standard IHD), with CVVH, replacement fluid is added directly to the blood and solute is removed by convection. One advantage of CVVH is that, as in peritoneal dialysis, the amount of urea clearance can be directly estimated from the total ultrafiltrate volume. This is because the urea nitrogen concentration of the ultrafiltrate will be essentially the same as the urea nitrogen concentration of plasma. A caveat here is that this will only be the case when the replacement fluid is added to the blood after the filter ("post-filter"), as depicted in Figure 11.2, but not if it is added "pre-filter."

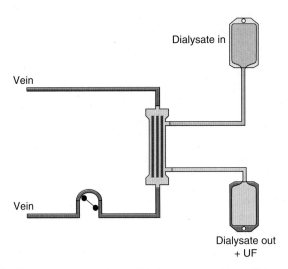

FIGURE 11.3 Continuous venovenous hemodialysis or sustained low-efficiency dialysis. (Adapted from Bellomo R, Ronco C, Mehta RL. Nomenclature for continuous renal replacement therapies. *Am J Kidney Dis.* 1996;28(5):S2–S7.)

Some trainees have difficulty understanding how hemofiltration cleans the blood. Let us say that you have been dyeing some clothes in the bathtub and the bathtub is now half-full of blue water. You are instructed to clean the water without altering the level of the bathwater. This can be simply done by opening the drain to remove the blue water and running clear water into the tub at the same rate as the rate of water going down the drain. This is a homespun analogy for "isovolumic hemofiltration" (see Patient 4).

PATIENT 4

A 70-kg male patient with sepsis, hypotension, and oliguric AKI is started on CVVH. The prescription is for 2 L of replacement fluid to be given hourly with 2 L/h of total ultrafiltration, that is, no net ultrafiltration or "isovolumic hemofiltration." Both the plasma and ultrafiltrate urea nitrogen concentrations are 50 mg/dL. What is the daily clearance?

Since similar to peritoneal dialysis, the total fluid removed (total ultrafiltrate) contains urea at approximately the same concentration as that found in the plasma, the clearance can be taken to be the total ultrafiltration rate. From a number of studies, we know that 20 mL/kg/h is an adequate dose of CVVH. In this case, we have 2 L/70 kg/h = 28.6 mL/kg/h, which is adequate.

Now let us assume that the patient is fluid overloaded, and the goal is to remove 2.4 L (100 mL/h) of extra fluid daily from the patient. The total ultrafiltration will now be 48 L + 2.4 L = 50.4 L, and the "net ultrafiltration" will be 2.4 L (be careful not to confuse total with net ultrafiltration!). Now the dose of CVVH is 2.1 L/70 kg/h = 30 mL/kg/h, slightly more than with isovolumic hemofiltration.

With CVVHD, as with dialytic ultrafiltration using IHD, the concentration of urea nitrogen will be somewhat lower in the ultrafiltrate than in the plasma. This is because during dialysis, urea is predominantly removed by diffusion rather than convection, and there is some residual concentration gradient between the plasma and the dialysate. Thus, providing replacement fluid is given "post-filter," CVVH is somewhat more efficient in removing solute than CVVHD (this is not the case if the replacement fluid is given "pre-filter," which is frequently done in practice). CVVHDF will result in the greatest urea clearance, but is not really necessary, as it is easy to achieve adequate clearance with CVVH or CVVHD alone. Since "middle-molecular-weight" solutes (i.e., 500–5,000 Da) such as cytokines are removed better by convection rather than diffusion, some favor CVVH over CVVHD in inflamed/septic patients, though there is no proof that CVVH results in better outcomes than any other modality of renal replacement therapy in critically ill patients.

References

Cooper BA, Branley P, Bulfone L, et al. A randomized, controlled trial of early versus late initiation of dialysis. *N Engl J Med.* 2010;363:609–619.

Lubowitz H, Slatopolsky E, Shankel S, et al. Glomerular filtration rate. Determination in patients with chronic renal disease. *JAMA.* 1967;199(4):252–256.

Selected Readings

Daugirdas JT. Physiologic principles and urea kinetic modeling. In: Daugirdas JT, Blake P, Ing TS, eds. *Handbook of Dialysis.* 5th ed. Philadelphia, PA: Wolters Kluwer/Lippincott Williams & Wilkins; 2015.

Teo BW, Messer JS, Chua HR, et al. Continuous renal replacement therapies. In: Daugirdas JT, Blake P, Ing TS, eds. *Handbook of Dialysis.* 5th ed. Philadelphia, PA: Wolters Kluwer/Lippincott Williams & Wilkins; 2015.

When Does Metabolic Acidosis Require Treatment with Bicarbonate?

12

Administration of bicarbonate in patients with metabolic acidosis is an area of medicine that has resulted in some confusion for trainees over the past few decades. In the 1970s, it was really not much of a debatable issue; at that time, it was widely accepted that bicarbonate was a cornerstone of therapy in virtually all patients with metabolic acidosis, including those with lactic acidosis and ketoacidosis, and was a first-line therapy after cardiac arrest. In more recent times, bicarbonate therapy has become more nuanced. As with the approach to correction of hyponatremia (Chapter 7), the approach to correction of metabolic acidosis is very dependent on the clinical context. Type and severity of metabolic acidosis are very important considerations, as are coexisting electrolyte abnormalities.

Hyperchloremic (non–anion gap) acidosis is due to either loss of bicarbonate or gain of nonvolatile acid with resulting titration of bicarbonate. The kidney retains chloride to maintain electroneutrality. Hyperchloremic acidosis should generally be treated with bicarbonate or other alkali, unless the cause is expected to be self-limited. For example, with acute diarrhea or prerenal failure, it may not be necessary to give bicarbonate, as the metabolic acidosis will likely correct on its own once the underlying problem is rectified. However, there should be little disagreement about the importance of treating chronic metabolic acidosis in patients with chronic kidney disease (CKD). In such patients, metabolic acidosis is not expected to improve on its own. Accumulating data indicate that correction of even mild renal acidosis has many beneficial effects, such as improved nitrogen balance and possibly delayed progression of CKD (de Brito-Ashurst et al., 2009; Mahajan et al., 2010; Phisitkul et al., 2010). Another clear-cut indication for alkali therapy is renal tubular acidosis (RTA), where alkali therapy can prevent permanent complications such as bone disease (Morris and Sebastian, 2002).

A different situation exists with high anion gap acidosis. Most of these disorders are due to overproduction of an organic acid, most commonly lactic acid or ketoacids. For instance, in lactic acidosis, the decrease in serum bicarbonate concentration is directly related to the amount of lactic acid production:

$$H^+lactate^- + HCO_3^- \rightarrow H_2O + CO_2 + Lactate^-$$

Accumulation of the lactate ion occurs if its rate of production outpaces the rate of urinary excretion plus metabolism. If and when it is metabolized, however, lactate will generate bicarbonate. If lactic acid production diminishes after successful treatment of the underlying disease (e.g., septic shock), the acidosis should correct on its own. Therefore, the role of exogenous bicarbonate therapy in patients with lactic acidosis is controversial (Stacpoole, 1986; Kraut and Madias, 2012). Severe acidemia (pH <7.1) may produce hemodynamic instability because of reduced left ventricular contractility, arterial vasodilation, and impaired responsiveness to catecholamines (Mitchell et al., 1972). However, experimental studies indicate that an increase in systemic pH engendered by bicarbonate therapy can be accompanied by worsening of intracellular acidosis (due to increased production of CO_2 with diffusion of CO_2 into cells). This dissociation between systemic and intracellular pH is most evident in patients with circulatory failure (Weil et al., 1986). Rapid infusion of sodium bicarbonate may increase the PCO_2 (especially in patients with impaired alveolar gas exchange), accelerate the production of lactic acid (due to worsening intracellular acidosis leading to increased anaerobic metabolism), lower the ionized calcium (due to a rapid rise in systemic pH which will increase the number of negative charges on albumin and thus the amount of calcium that is bound to albumin), expand the extracellular space (due to the sodium administered), and raise the serum sodium concentration resulting in hypernatremia (when hypertonic solutions are employed).

There are only a few small randomized studies of bicarbonate therapy in lactic acidosis, and these were done over 20 years ago. In a crossover study, 14 patients with lactic acidosis (serum HCO_3 <17 mEq/L and arterial lactate >2.5 mEq/L) in a single intensive care unit (ICU) received, in random order, 2 mmol/kg of sodium bicarbonate or an equivalent dose of sodium chloride (Cooper et al., 1990). Bicarbonate therapy produced a significant rise in arterial pH and serum HCO_3, but there were no differences in cardiac output, mean arterial pressure, or pulmonary capillary wedge pressure. In another randomized crossover trial of 10 patients with lactic acidosis comparing sodium bicarbonate (1 mmol/kg) and an equivalent dose of sodium chloride, bicarbonate therapy again significantly increased the arterial pH and serum bicarbonate, but again there was no hemodynamic benefit of bicarbonate (Mathieu et al., 1991).

So which patients with lactic acidosis should get bicarbonate therapy? The answer is really not known. It has been suggested that patients with lactic acidosis and severe acidemia (i.e., pH <7.1 and plasma HCO_3 ≤6 mEq/L) receive bicarbonate therapy. This is particularly the case if the pH cannot be further increased by increasing ventilation. This recommendation is based on physiologic principles and not clinical trials, and thus not evidence-based. It should be stressed, however, that in the small clinical trials cited previously that failed to show a clinically important benefit of bicarbonate therapy, arterial pH was higher than 7.1. It is possible that bicarbonate therapy would affect outcomes when the pH is lower than 7.1.

Another concern about bicarbonate therapy is that it can lead to a decrease in cerebrospinal fluid (CSF) pH by two different mechanisms: (1) an increase in local PCO_2 in the brain and CSF and (2) slow entry of bicarbonate into the CSF. Because CSF bicarbonate concentration does not rise as rapidly as the CSF PCO_2, "paradoxical" CSF acidemia can result and may be associated with neurologic deterioration (Posner and Plum, 1967). CSF acidemia provides a persistent stimulus for hyperventilation even in the event that systemic pH is increased by bicarbonate therapy. Very rapid increases in systemic pH may thus occur when bicarbonate is administered. With very severe acidosis (i.e., serum bicarbonate concentration <4 mEq/L), relatively small bicarbonate concentration changes will have a great impact on arterial pH. This is due to the nonlinear relationship between pH and HCO_3 (see *Patient 1*).

PATIENT 1

A 75-year-old man is "found down" in his apartment after the neighbors became alarmed that they had not seen him for many days and called 911. He is admitted to the ICU with obtundation. He is thought to have sepsis and given broad-spectrum antibiotics and pressors. A nephrologist is asked to dialyze him because of oliguric acute kidney injury (AKI) and severe acidosis. Serum chemistries reveal urea nitrogen 180 mg/dL, creatinine 18 mg/dL, sodium 131 mmol/L, potassium 7 mmol/L, chloride

100 mmol/L, total carbon dioxide 1 mmol/L, total calcium 9 mg/dL, inorganic phosphorus 16 mg/dL, total magnesium 2 mg/dL, and albumin 4 g/dL. Arterial blood gas (ABG) reveal pH 6.8, Pco_2 7 mm Hg, and HCO_3 1 mmol/L.

Scenario 1: After 2 hours of dialysis, the patient codes and dies. But immediately prior to the code a repeat ABG had been obtained per order of the nephrologist, which reveals:

$$\text{ABG: pH} > 7.7 \text{ (off the scale), } Pco_2 \text{ 10 mm Hg, and}$$
$$HCO_3 \text{ 20 mmol/L}$$

How is this possible? Remember Henderson's equation:

$$[H^+] = (24 \times Pco_2)/[HCO_3]$$

In this case,

$$[H^+] = (24 \times 10)/20 = 12$$

Since pH = $-\log[H^+]$, for every twofold change in $[H^+]$, pH will change by 0.3 units (Table 12.1). When $[H^+] = 40$, pH is 7.4. When $[H^+] = 20$, pH is 7.7. Therefore, when $[H^+] = 12$, pH will be nearly 8.0 (off the scale).

It can be seen from Henderson's equation that small absolute changes in bicarbonate concentration will have a large effect on pH when bicarbonate concentration is very low. Note the Pco_2 did not change much in this patient as there is continued hyperventilation due to paradoxical CSF acidemia.

Scenario 2: Fortunately, Scenario 1 did not really happen. The house staff had started a bicarbonate infusion and raised the plasma bicarbonate concentration to 10 mmol/L before dialysis was started. A repeat ABG just prior to dialysis showed:

$$\text{ABG: pH 7.42, } Pco_2 \text{ 16 mm Hg, and } HCO_3 \text{ 10 mmol/L}$$

TABLE 12.1	Relationship between pH and Hydrogen Ion Concentration
pH	**[H⁺]**
7.1	80
7.2	63
7.3	51
7.4	40
7.5	32
7.6	25
7.7	20

You can check that these numbers are right from Henderson's equation:

$$[H^+] = (24 \times Pco_2)/HCO_3 = (24 \times 16)/10$$
$$= 38 \text{ (therefore, pH is 7.42)}$$

Now after 2 hours of dialysis:

ABG: pH 7.62, Pco_2 20 mm Hg, and HCO_3 20 mmol/L

$$[H^+] = (24 \times Pco_2)/[HCO_3] = (24 \times 20)/20$$
$$= 24 \text{ (therefore, pH is indeed 7.62)}$$

This is still high, but at least compatible with life.

In this patient, the cause of extreme metabolic acidosis was attributed to renal failure alone, as an extensive search for another cause of high anion gap acidosis including tests for both L-lactate and D-lactate, beta-hydroxybutyrate, ethylene glycol, methanol, salicylate, acetaminophen, metformin, and 5-oxoproline all were negative. In severe renal failure, retention of both hydrogen ions and anions such as sulfate, phosphate, and urate can rarely result in a very marked anion gap acidosis.

Appropriate bicarbonate therapy may have been life-saving in this patient (indeed immediate dialysis may have been lethal due to too rapid correction of pH!). There are other situations where bicarbonate therapy itself can be potentially lethal, particularly when metabolic acidosis coexists with hypokalemia. This is because administration of bicarbonate will shift potassium into cells (by both pH-dependent and pH-independent or ionic mechanisms), thus lowering plasma potassium levels (Fraley and Adler, 1977). In addition, if hypocalcemia is present, administering bicarbonate and raising systemic pH will increase the number of anionic binding sites on albumin and lead to an increase in the albumin-bound fraction and a decrease in ionized calcium (Schaer, 1976). A sudden decrease in ionized calcium, especially if it is already low to start with, can cause tetany and seizures. Most experienced nephrologists have witnessed this more than once.

PATIENT 2

A 40-year-old alcoholic woman is admitted with abdominal pain, nausea, and vomiting. Physical examination reveals muscle wasting, flat neck veins, and decreased skin turgor, suggesting malnutrition and volume depletion. Serum chemistries reveal urea nitrogen 8 mg/dL, creatinine 0.8 mg/dL, sodium 135 mmol/L, potassium 3.4 mmol/L, chloride 100 mmol/L, total carbon dioxide 5 mmol/L, glucose 70 mg/dL, total calcium

9 mg/dL, inorganic phosphorus 3.0 mg/dL, total magnesium 1.8 mg/dL, and albumin 3.0 g/dL. ABG reveal pH 7.1, Pco_2 17 mm Hg, and HCO_3 5 mmol/L. Serum ethanol was undetectable. A medical resident, alarmed by the severe acidosis and cognizant of volume depletion and mild hypoglycemia, administered isotonic sodium bicarbonate in 5% dextrose at a rate of 250 mL/h. Thiamine was also administered. Four hours after the beginning of the intravenous infusion, the patient suffered a cardiac arrest and could not be resuscitated.

What happened here? (As opposed to the "death" in Patient 1, this patient really did expire.) Patient 2 also had a high anion gap metabolic acidosis, with an uncorrected anion gap of 30 mEq/L (it was actually a little higher when corrected for the low serum albumin, since albumin normally accounts for about half of the anion gap) (Feldman et al., 2005). Urinalysis in this patient showed ketonuria without glycosuria and the serum beta-hydroxybutyrate was elevated. These findings are consistent with alcoholic ketoacidosis.

Alcoholic ketoacidosis typically occurs in malnourished patients with chronic alcoholism after binge alcohol ingestion. When they present to the hospital, blood ethanol levels are typically low or not detectable since alcohol ingestion has ceased. Increased levels of catecholamines and cortisol resulting from alcohol withdrawal combined with the hormonal responses to fasting (low insulin and high glucagon levels) cause a marked increase in lipolysis, fatty acid delivery to the liver, and ketogenesis. Hypoglycemia or hyperglycemia, hypokalemia, hypophosphatemia, and hypomagnesemia are common.

Hypokalemia in alcoholic ketoacidosis is due to both decreased dietary intake and increased renal loss in conjunction with ketoacid anions. Secondary hyperaldosteronism from volume depletion (due to poor intake and vomiting) also will contribute to renal potassium loss. Ketoacidosis can usually be at least partially corrected by administration of saline in dextrose solutions. However, dextrose solutions should be avoided in patients with hypokalemia since they stimulate insulin secretion, increasing cellular potassium intake and worsening hypokalemia. Administration of sodium bicarbonate is not necessary in this condition and will lead to further translocation of potassium into cells (Fraley and Adler, 1977).

This patient likely died from a cardiac arrhythmia brought on by sudden worsening of hypokalemia caused by the intravenous infusion of isotonic bicarbonate in dextrose.

References

Cooper DJ, Walley KR, Wiggs BR, et al. Bicarbonate does not improve hemodynamics in critically ill patients who have lactic acidosis. A prospective, controlled clinical study. *Ann Intern Med.* 1990;112:492.

de Brito-Ashurst I, Varagunam M, Raftery MJ, et al. Bicarbonate supplementation slows progression of CKD and improves nutritional status. *J Am Soc Nephrol.* 2009;20:2075.

Feldman M, Soni N, Dickson B. Influence of hypoalbuminemia or hyperalbuminemia on the serum anion gap. *J Lab Clin Med.* 2005;146(6):317.

Fraley DS, Adler S. Correction of hyperkalemia by bicarbonate despite constant blood pH. *Kidney Int.* 1977;12(5):354–360.

Kraut JA, Madias NE. Treatment of acute metabolic acidosis: a pathophysiologic approach. *Nat Rev Nephrol.* 2012;8:589.

Mahajan A, Simoni J, Sheather SJ, et al. Daily oral sodium bicarbonate preserves glomerular filtration rate by slowing its decline in early hypertensive nephropathy. *Kidney Int.* 2010;78:303.

Mathieu D, Neviere R, Billard V, et al. Effects of bicarbonate therapy on hemodynamics and tissue oxygenation in patients with lactic acidosis: a prospective, controlled clinical study. *Crit Care Med.* 1991;19:1352.

Mitchell JH, Wildenthal K, Johnson RL Jr. The effects of acid–base disturbances on cardiovascular and pulmonary function. *Kidney Int.* 1972;1:375.

Morris RC Jr, Sebastian A. Alkali therapy in renal tubular acidosis: who needs it? *J Am Soc Nephrol.* 2002;13:2186.

Phisitkul S, Khanna A, Simoni J, et al. Amelioration of metabolic acidosis in patients with low GFR reduced kidney endothelin production and kidney injury, and better preserved GFR. *Kidney Int.* 2010;77:617.

Posner JB, Plum F. Spinal-fluid pH and neurologic symptoms in systemic acidosis. *N Engl J Med.* 1967;277:605.

Schaer H. Effects on ionized calcium of a correction of acidosis with alkalinizing agents. A rational basis for the administration of calcium in cardiac resuscitation. *Br J Anaesth.* 1976;48(4):327–332.

Stacpoole PW. Lactic acidosis: the case against bicarbonate therapy. *Ann Intern Med.* 1986;105:276.

Weil MH, Rackow EC, Trevino R, et al. Difference in acid–base state between venous and arterial blood during cardiopulmonary resuscitation. *N Engl J Med.* 1986;315:153.

Is There Any Advantage to Colloids versus Crystalloids for Volume Repletion?

Rapid volume repletion is indicated in patients with severe hypovolemic or septic shock, as a delay in therapy can result in ischemic injury and possibly irreversible shock and multiorgan system failure. Various monitoring methods have been used to guide fluid resuscitation. Classically, pressure measurements such as central venous pressure or pulmonary capillary wedge pressure were employed. More recently, volume measurements such as inferior vena cava diameter using echocardiography or bedside ultrasound have been more frequently used. Some data suggest that respiratory variation in the arterial pressure tracing can be used to estimate the adequacy of fluid resuscitation, with large stroke volume or pulse pressure variations suggesting persistent hypovolemia and right ventricular underfilling (Gunn and Pinsky, 2001; Magder, 2004). The use of stroke volume or pulse pressure variation to assess volume responsiveness requires that the patient be mechanically ventilated (Soubrier et al., 2007). Other noninvasive tests, such as hemodynamic response to positional changes and leg raising, have also been employed (Monnet et al., 2006).

There are three major classes of replacement fluids:

- Crystalloid solutions—isotonic or "normal" saline, buffered solutions (e.g., Ringer lactate, bicarbonate-buffered 0.45% saline, i.e., 75 mmol/L sodium bicarbonate added to 0.45% saline), and chloride-restrictive fluids (e.g., Hartmann solution)
- Colloid-containing solutions—albumin solutions, hyperoncotic starch, dextran, and gelatin

95

- Blood products or substitutes—packed red cells and blood substitutes

What is "normal saline"? It is actually "normal physiologic saline" or more meaningfully "isotonic saline." It is 0.9% saline, which means that there are 0.9 g of sodium chloride (NaCl) per deciliter (100 mL) of water, or 9 g/L. The molecular weight of sodium chloride is approximately 58.5 g/mol (remember that a mole is the molecular weight in grams, and a millimole is the molecular weight in milligrams). To convert 9 g/L to mmol/L, divide by the molecular weight (58.5 g/mol), which gives 0.154 mol/L (154 mmol/L). Since NaCl dissociates into two ions, sodium and chloride, 154 mmol/L NaCl = 154 mmol/L of Na^+ and 154 mmol/L of Cl^-. Since both sodium and chloride are univalent, 154 mmol/L = 154 mEq/L for both ions. Note that one cannot technically say NaCl 154 mEq/L, as mEq/L is used only for charged substances (ions) and sodium chloride is uncharged.

One might expect the osmolality of normal saline to be 154 × 2 = 308 mmol/L, but this is not the case. One must take into account the osmotic coefficient, a correction for nonideal solutions. The osmotic coefficient of NaCl is 0.93; therefore, the osmolality of a 0.9% saline solution is 154 × 2 × 0.93 = 286 mmol/L, which is isotonic (or iso-osmolar).

How about *albumin solutions*? Whether or not one gives iso-oncotic (5%) albumin or hyperoncotic (25%) albumin, the osmolality is dependent on the sodium and chloride concentrations (which vary from 130 to 160 mmol/L depending on the manufacturer). Remember that osmolality is a measure of the number of particles per unit volume and thus smaller molecular weight substances will count just as much as large ones. Albumin is very large compared to electrolytes—the molecular weight of albumin is about 70,000 Da—so in a 5% albumin solution, the albumin contributes only a small portion of the total osmolality:

$$5\% = 5 \text{ g}/100 \text{ mL or } 50 \text{ g/L} \times 1 \text{ mol}/70{,}000 \text{ g}$$
$$= 0.0007 \text{ mol/L} = 0.7 \text{ mmol/L}$$

Even 25% albumin contains only about 0.7 × 5 = 3.5 mmol/L. This is why the electrolytes need to be added—otherwise the solution would be dangerously hypotonic and could cause hemolysis. So when you are administering albumin, you are not giving albumin alone but rather albumin in (approximately) isotonic saline.

The choice of replacement fluid depends in part upon the type of fluid that needs to be replaced. Blood transfusion for hemorrhage/blood loss and plasma products for coagulopathy are self-evident and will not be further discussed. The focus will be on the ongoing colloid (usually albumin) versus crystalloid debate.

IS THERE A ROLE FOR ALBUMIN INFUSIONS RATHER THAN CRYSTALLOID INFUSIONS?

In general, crystalloids are preferred over colloid-containing solutions in patients with volume depletion not due to bleeding. This is because studies have shown that saline solutions are as effective as other crystalloid solutions and colloid-containing solutions, and are much less expensive (Finfer et al., 2004; Annane et al., 2013). Hyperoncotic starch solutions should not be used because of an increased risk of acute kidney injury, need for renal replacement therapy, and mortality (Zarychanski et al., 2013).

Since crystalloids will distribute into the extracellular fluid whereas colloids will primarily stay in the intravascular space, up to three times as much saline as colloid must be administered to cause a similar increase in plasma volume (McIlroy and Kharasch, 2003). This may be an advantage of crystalloids if interstitial fluid deficits are also present, but crystalloids may lead to more peripheral edema in other circumstances (Zarins et al., 1978).

Because of the relatively high permeability of the alveolar capillaries to albumin, colloid administration leads to a higher interstitial oncotic pressure in the lungs than in subcutaneous tissue (Taylor, 1981). If hypoalbuminemia is present, there is a parallel reduction in alveolar interstitial albumin concentration, since less albumin moves across the capillary wall, and thus little tendency to the development of pulmonary edema (Zarins et al., 1978). This differs from the effect of hypoalbuminemia on the development of peripheral edema. However, rapid colloid infusion can indeed precipitate pulmonary edema in some hypoalbuminemic patients, such as those with severe nephrotic syndrome (Reid et al., 1996). This is due to a rapid increase in plasma volume with a resulting increase in pulmonary capillary hydrostatic pressure.

The safety of colloids was first questioned in a meta-analysis performed by Velanovich (1989). Since that time, there have been a number of meta-analyses that have also questioned the safety and efficacy of colloids. The largest one reported no difference in outcome for patients treated with albumin versus crystalloids (Wilkes, 2001).

There is some evidence favoring the use of colloids for the treatment of hypovolemic shock. In a multicenter, open-label trial (CRISTAL), 2,857 patients with hypovolemic shock due to any cause were randomly assigned to resuscitation with intravenous crystalloid or colloid solutions (Annane et al., 2013). There was no difference in 28-day mortality or need for renal replacement therapy between the groups, but patients treated with colloids had slightly less days on the ventilator and on vasopressors and a slightly lower 90-day mortality (31% vs. 34%). These findings are not convincing enough to favor the use of colloids for this indication. In a multicenter randomized trial of nearly 7,000 hypovolemic medical and surgical ICU patients, entitled the SAFE (Saline versus Albumin Fluid Evaluation) trial, fluid resuscitation using either 4% albumin solution or isotonic saline was compared (Finfer et al., 2004). All-cause mortality at 28 days (the primary end point of the study), multiorgan failure, the duration of hospitalization, and effect upon systemic pH were similar in both groups (SAFE Study Investigators et al., 2011).

IS THERE ANY ADVANTAGE OF LACTATED RINGER OVER ISOTONIC SALINE?

Large-volume resuscitation using isotonic saline may be associated with the development of hyperchloremic metabolic acidosis, sometimes called dilutional acidosis (Mirza et al., 1999). This has led to suggestions that physiologically buffered fluids (e.g., lactated Ringer solution or 0.45% saline solution with 75 mmol/L of sodium bicarbonate) be used instead of isotonic saline for large-volume resuscitation, though there are no data to support this contention. Chloride-restrictive fluids such as lactated Hartmann solution have also been advocated, since hyperchloremic solutions are associated with an increased risk of acute kidney injury due to increased renal vasoconstriction and decreased glomerular filtration (Krajewski et al., 2015). These studies unfortunately have major design flaws that limit their applicability to clinical practice. The composition of intravenous solutions commonly used in clinical practice is given in Table 13.1.

TABLE 13.1	Composition of Commonly Used Intravenous Fluids					
Solution	Sodium	Potassium	Chloride	Bicarbonate	Lactate	Calcium
0.9% saline	154	0	154	0	0	0
Lactated Ringer	130	4	109	0	28	3
5% albumin	130–160	<1	130–160	0	0	0
0.45% saline/ 75 mmol sodium bicarbonate	152	0	77	75	0	0

All values are in mEq/L (mEq/L = mmol/L for all analytes except for calcium, which is divalent, for which 3 mEq/L = 1.5 mmol/L).

HOW MUCH VOLUME SHOULD BE GIVEN IN SEPTIC SHOCK?

Early "goal-directed therapy," using physiologic measures of adequate volume resuscitation, has reported mean infusion volumes in the first 6 hours of 3 to 5 L in septic patients (Rivers et al., 2001), though later trials have reported mean infusion volumes of 2 to 3 L (ARISE Investigators et al., 2014; ProCESS Investigators et al., 2014). Thus, rapid, large-volume infusions of intravenous fluids appear to be beneficial in severe sepsis or septic shock, unless there is clinical or radiographic evidence of heart failure. However, it is crucial that fluid administration be stopped if pulmonary edema ensues or if it is not providing clinical benefit, and patients receiving aggressive fluid repletion require close monitoring in an ICU setting. Once patients are fluid resuscitated, a continued liberal approach to intravenous fluid administration has been shown to prolong the duration of mechanical ventilation when compared to a more restrictive approach accompanied by diuretic administration (National Heart, Lung, and Blood Institute Acute Respiratory Distress Syndrome (ARDS) Clinical Trials Network et al., 2006). There is no greater benefit of colloids versus crystalloids in septic shock, and there is potential harm from using starch rather than a crystalloid solution (Perner et al., 2012; Caironi et al., 2014).

PATIENT 1

A 50-year-old male is admitted to the ICU with fever, hypotension, and decreased urine output, and is diagnosed to have septic shock. His chest radiograph shows clear lung fields. He is treated with broad-spectrum antibiotics and intravenous fluids.

Q: Which of the following fluid regimens is most appropriate in this patient?

1. Intravenous saline 2 to 3 L given rapidly with close observation
2. Intravenous saline 250 mL/h
3. Intravenous 5% albumin 250 mL/h
4. Intravenous 25% albumin 250 mL bolus

A: The correct answer is intravenous saline 2 to 3 L given rapidly with close observation. If the patient remains hypotensive, and there is no sign of fluid overload as determined by chest radiograph and either central venous pressure monitoring or ultrasound assessment of intravascular volume, additional fluid resuscitation can be considered. There is no role for albumin in the management of septic shock.

PATIENT 2

A 75-year-old male anuric ESRD (end-stage renal disease) patient is admitted to the ICU with sepsis. He is hypotensive and weighs 50 kg. He receives 16 L of isotonic saline, after which his serum bicarbonate decreases from 25 to 10 mEq/L and the serum chloride increases from 103 to 115 mEq/L. The anion gap increases by 5 mEq/L.

Q: What is the nature of the metabolic acidosis?

A: The bicarbonate space (BS) can be estimated to be 50% of the body weight, which in this case is 50 kg $\times$ 0.5 = 25 L. After receiving 16 L of saline, the body bicarbonate would now be distributed in 41 L instead of 25 L, diluting the concentration as follows:

$$\text{Initial BS (25 L)} \times \text{Initial serum } [HCO_3^-] \text{ (25 mEq/L)}$$
$$= \text{Final BS (41 L)} \times \text{Final serum } [HCO_3^-]$$

Final serum $[HCO_3^-]$ = 625/41 = 15 mEq/L. The increase in anion gap (presumably due to production of lactic acid with lactate accumulation) accounts for the further 5-mEq/L decrease in serum $[HCO_3^-]$.

References

Annane D, Siami S, Jaber S, et al. Effects of fluid resuscitation with colloids vs crystalloids on mortality in critically ill patients presenting with hypovolemic shock: the CRISTAL randomized trial. *JAMA.* 2013;310:1809–1817.

ARISE Investigators, ANZICS Clinical Trials Group, Peake SL, et al. Goal-directed resuscitation for patients with early septic shock. *N Engl J Med.* 2014;371:1496–1506.

Caironi P, Tognoni G, Masson S, et al. Albumin replacement in patients with severe sepsis or septic shock. *N Engl J Med.* 2014;370:1412–1421.

Finfer S, Bellomo R, Boyce N, et al. A comparison of albumin and saline for fluid resuscitation in the intensive care unit. *N Engl J Med.* 2004;350:2247–2256.

Gunn SR, Pinsky MR. Implications of arterial pressure variation in patients in the intensive care unit. *Curr Opin Crit Care.* 2001;7:212–217.

Krajewski ML, Raghunathan K, Paluszkiewicz SM, et al. Meta-analysis of high- versus low-chloride content in perioperative and critical care fluid resuscitation. *Br J Surg.* 2015;102:24–36.

Magder S. Clinical usefulness of respiratory variations in arterial pressure. *Am J Respir Crit Care Med.* 2004;169:151–155.

McIlroy DR, Kharasch ED. Acute intravascular volume expansion with rapidly administered crystalloid or colloid in the setting of moderate hypovolemia. *Anesth Analg.* 2003;96:1572–1577.

Mirza BI, Sahani M, Leehey DJ, et al. Saline-induced dilutional acidosis in a maintenance hemodialysis patient. *Int J Artif Organs.* 1999;22(10):676–678.

Monnet X, Rienzo M, Osman D, et al. Passive leg raising predicts fluid responsiveness in the critically ill. *Crit Care Med.* 2006;34:1402–1407.

National Heart, Lung, and Blood Institute Acute Respiratory Distress Syndrome (ARDS) Clinical Trials Network, Wheeler AP, Bernard GR, et al. Pulmonary-artery versus central venous catheter to guide treatment of acute lung injury. *N Engl J Med*. 2006;354:2213–2224.

Perner A, Haase N, Guttormsen AB, et al. Hydroxyethyl starch 130/0.42 versus Ringer's acetate in severe sepsis. *N Engl J Med*. 2012;367:124–134.

ProCESS Investigators, Yealy DM, Kellum JA, et al. A randomized trial of protocol-based care for early septic shock. *N Engl J Med*. 2014;370:1683–1693.

Reid CJ, Marsh MJ, Murdoch IM, et al. Nephrotic syndrome in childhood complicated by life threatening pulmonary oedema. *BMJ*. 1996;312(7022):36–38.

Rivers E, Nguyen B, Havstad S, et al. Early goal-directed therapy in the treatment of severe sepsis and septic shock. *N Engl J Med*. 2001;345:1368–1377.

SAFE Study Investigators, Finfer S, McEvoy S, et al. Impact of albumin compared to saline on organ function and mortality of patients with severe sepsis. *Intensive Care Med*. 2011;37:86–96.

Soubrier S, Saulnier F, Hubert H, et al. Can dynamic indicators help the prediction of fluid responsiveness in spontaneously breathing critically ill patients? *Intensive Care Med*. 2007;33: 1117–1124.

Taylor AE. Capillary fluid filtration. Starling forces and lymph flow. *Circ Res*. 1981;49:557–575.

Velanovich V. Crystalloid versus colloid fluid resuscitation: a meta-analysis of mortality. *Surgery*. 1989;105:65–71.

Wilkes MM, Navickis RJ. Patient survival after human albumin administration: a meta-analysis of randomized, controlled trials. *Ann Intern Med*. 2001;135:149–164.

Zarins CK, Rice CL, Peters RM, et al. Lymph and pulmonary response to isobaric reduction in plasma oncotic pressure in baboons. *Circ Res*. 1978;43:925–930.

Zarychanski R, Abou-Setta AM, Turgeon AF, et al. Association of hydroxyethyl starch administration with mortality and acute kidney injury in critically ill patients requiring volume resuscitation: a systematic review and meta-analysis. *JAMA*. 2013;309:678–688.

14

Is Computed Tomography with Contrast or Magnetic Resonance Imaging with Contrast Preferred in Patients with Chronic Kidney Disease?

This is a clinical question that keeps coming up on nephrology rounds. Radiocontrast-induced nephropathy is a real concern in patients with risk factors for this complication. The most important risk factor is the presence and degree of underlying chronic kidney disease (CKD). In the past, magnetic resonance imaging (MRI) was generally chosen as an alternative to computed tomography (CT) when kidney disease was present, as it was thought that MRI contrast agents, including gadolinium, were safe in CKD. This all changed with the discovery of nephrogenic systemic fibrosis (NSF) in the late 1990s and the probable role of gadolinium in its pathogenesis, as gadolinium deposits have been found in tissue specimens from patients with NSF. NSF is relatively rare but serious disease, with an unremitting course and high morbidity and mortality (Mendoza et al., 2006).

RADIOCONTRAST NEPHROPATHY

Epidemiology

Radiocontrast nephropathy is a generally reversible form of acute kidney injury (AKI) that occurs soon after the administration of radiocontrast media (Rudnick et al., 1994). As the pathogenesis is difficult to study in humans, most of our understanding of the mechanisms of radiocontrast nephropathy derives from animal models. AKI results from a combination of renal vasoconstriction resulting in medullary hypoxia (possibly mediated by alterations in nitric oxide, endothelin, and/or adenosine) and direct cytotoxic effects of the contrast agents (Persson et al., 2005). Inhibitors of both nitric oxide and prostaglandins cause marked ischemia and tubular necrosis in the medullary thick ascending limb of the loop of Henle in rats exposed to radiocontrast (Agmon et al., 1994). The outer medulla appears particularly susceptible to contrast-induced reduction in renal blood flow because of the relative hypoxic conditions in this nephron segment (Heyman et al., 2005). Direct tubular injury is associated with generation of oxygen free radicals, which has led to numerous studies evaluating a possible apparent protective effect of N-acetylcysteine (NAC) as well as trials of bicarbonate therapy to prevent nephropathy.

Incidence

The reported incidence of radiocontrast-induced nephropathy varies widely, depending on the presence or absence of patient risk factors, the most important being CKD. Other patient risk factors include age, diabetes, decreased renal blood flow from any cause (such as hypovolemia, hypotension, heart failure, cirrhosis), and possibly multiple myeloma (Table 14.1). The most important modifiable risk factors are dose of contrast and the presence of hypovolemia. In patients with no risk factors, for example, a young nondiabetic patient, the risk of radiocontrast nephropathy is negligible (<1%), but very high-risk patients, for example, an older diabetic patient with severe CKD, the risk may be 30% or greater.

TABLE 14.1	Risk Factors for Contrast-Induced Nephropathy

Age
CKD
Diabetes, if CKD present
Decreased renal blood flow from any cause (hypovolemia, hypotension, heart failure, cirrhosis, non-steroidal anti-inflammatory drugs)
Multiple myeloma?
Hyperglycemia (without diabetes)

CKD and Diabetes

The increase in risk with CKD is likely linearly related to the glomerular filtration rate (GFR). Among patients with CKD, diabetic patients are at higher risk for radiocontrast nephropathy compared with nondiabetic patients. In one prospective study, in patients with CKD (serum creatinine >1.7 mg/dL [150 μmol/L]) undergoing CT scan with contrast, diabetic patients had a greater than twofold higher incidence of radiocontrast nephropathy (8.8% vs. 4.0%, respectively) (Parfrey et al., 1989). Similarly, in an analysis of data from a randomized trial that included 250 patients with serum creatinine more than 1.5 mg/dL (133 μmol/L) who received iohexol during percutaneous coronary interventions, diabetic patients had a much higher incidence than controls (33% vs. 12%, respectively); however, diabetes did not increase the risk in patients without CKD (Rudnick et al., 1995).

Hyperglycemia

The degree of hyperglycemia may increase the risk for radiocontrast nephropathy in nondiabetic patients. In a study of 6,358 patients undergoing angiography following myocardial infarction, the adjusted risk of radiocontrast nephropathy increased as glucose levels increased in nondiabetic patients, with greater than twofold risk when blood glucose was more than 200 mg/dL (Stolker et al., 2010). Interestingly, an association between hyperglycemia and risk of contrast nephropathy was not seen in diabetic patients.

Type of Radiocontrast Agent

It is clear that first-generation hyperosmolal ionic contrast agents increase the risk of AKI compared to nonionic low-osmolal or iso-osmolal agents (Rudnick et al., 1995). However, it is less clear whether there is any difference between low-osmolal and iso-osmolal agents, the latter of which is considerably more expensive. This is discussed further later in the chapter.

Specific Radiologic Procedure

The risk of radiocontrast nephropathy in patients undergoing percutaneous angiography, particularly coronary angiography, is substantially higher than that with contrast CT scans, though the dose used is generally higher as well (Weisbord et al., 2008). The incidence of AKI may also be higher for patients who receive contrast for a nonelective versus elective contrast CT (Mitchell et al., 2010). In a prospective study of 633 outpatients who underwent contrast CT in the emergency department of a tertiary care center, of whom only 2.4% had eGFR less than 60 mL/min/1.73 m^2, 11% developed AKI (defined as an increase in serum creatinine >0.5 mg/dL [44 μmol/L] or >25% within 2–7 days after contrast administration). Six patients (1%) developed severe AKI (increase in serum creatinine ≥3 mg/dL or need for dialysis). The relatively high incidence of AKI in this study may be due to lack of adjustment for comorbidities such as hypotension, hyperglycemia, or volume depletion, but does point to the possibility of increased risk in an emergency room population.

Clinical Features

Clinical manifestations such as oliguria or an increase in the serum creatinine are generally observed within 24 to 48 hours after contrast exposure. The majority of patients are nonoliguric, so the severity of AKI is usually determined by the extent of increase in the serum creatinine. Unlike other types of AKI, radiocontrast nephropathy is generally characterized by relatively rapid recovery of renal function, with the serum creatinine starting to decline within 3 to 7 days (Rudnick et al., 1994). The urinary sediment may show classic findings of acute tubular necrosis (ATN), that is, pigmented "muddy-brown" granular casts. If contrast is still present in the urine, it will cause a markedly increased specific gravity (~1.050) because of the heavy weight of iodine (the effect of contrast on osmolality is less marked). The fractional sodium excretion (FENa) is often less than 1% in patients with radiocontrast nephropathy, particularly in its early phase. This may indicate intrarenal vasoconstriction and/or be a reflection of the nonoliguric state, leading to a lower urinary sodium concentration.

The differential diagnosis includes other causes of renal tubular injury (ischemic or toxic), acute interstitial nephritis, renal atheroemboli (after angiography), and prerenal failure. Renal atheroembolism after angiography should be suspected if there are other embolic lesions (such as blue toes or livedo reticularis), transient eosinophilia and/or hypocomplementemia, delayed development of AKI, or failure to recover renal function.

Radiocontrast nephropathy generally has a good prognosis. Most patients recover renal function without need for dialysis. However, some patients, especially diabetic patients with severe underlying CKD (i.e., eGFR <30 mL/min/1.73 m^2), may require dialysis, which may be permanent in a small percentage of cases.

PREVENTION OF RADIOCONTRAST NEPHROPATHY

Type and Amount of Contrast Agent

The renal toxicity of contrast agents appears to be related to their osmolality. Ionic high-osmolal first-generation agents were associated with a high rate of nephrotoxicity and are no longer employed. Second-generation agents, such as iohexol, are nonionic monomers with a lower osmolality than high-osmolal radiocontrast media; however, they still have an increased osmolality compared with plasma. In addition, there is an ionic low-osmolal contrast agent (ioxaglate). The newest nonionic contrast agents are iso-osmolal, being dimers with an osmolality of approximately 290 mmol/kg (iodixanol, the first such agent, is available in the United States).

A variety of preventive measures may reduce the risk of contrast nephropathy (Asif and Epstein, 2004; Pannu et al., 2006). The first consideration is to avoid contrast entirely by use of an alternate imaging method such as ultrasonography, MRI, or CT scanning without radiocontrast agents. If contrast is essential, use of lower doses of contrast (Cigarroa et al., 1989; Marenzi et al., 2009) and avoidance of repetitive studies that are closely spaced (within 48–72 hours) decrease the risk. The relationship between dose and toxicity is demonstrated by the observation that very small amounts of radiocontrast ($<$10 mL) can be safely used in patients with very severe CKD for examination of poorly maturing arteriovenous fistulae (Kian et al., 2006). Reduction of contrast dose during coronary angiography can be achieved by avoiding ventriculography and the use of endovascular ultrasound and during peripheral vascular contrast procedures with the use of carbon dioxide angiography (usually in combination with small amounts of iodinated contrast).

Do iso-osmolal agents have a lower risk than low-osmolal agents? In the initial trial comparing iodixanol and iohexol in 129 high-risk patients with diabetes and CKD (mean serum creatinine 1.5 mg/dL [133 µmol/L]) undergoing angiography, iodixanol was associated with a significantly lower incidence of a more than 0.5 mg/dL (44 µmol/L) rise in serum creatinine (3% vs. 26%) (Aspelin et al., 2003). However, three much larger subsequent trials that compared iodixanol with two other nonionic low-osmolal contrast agents (ioversol and iopamidol) in patients with diabetic and nondiabetic CKD found no difference in the incidence of contrast nephropathy among the different agents (Solomon et al., 2007; Rudnick et al., 2008; Laskey et al., 2009). A meta-analysis of 16 randomized trials also suggested that iodixanol was associated with a reduction in risk among patients with CKD when compared with iohexol, but not when compared with other nonionic low-osmolal contrast agents (Reed et al., 2009). Therefore, there appears to be an adverse effect of iohexol rather than a beneficial effect of iodixanol. The recent American College of Cardiology/American Heart Association (ACC/AHA) guidelines on percutaneous coronary intervention recommended the use of either an iso-osmolal contrast agent or a low-molecular-weight contrast agent other than iohexol or ioxaglate (Kushner et al., 2009).

Prophylaxis

The standard prophylactic measure when contrast is administered is intravenous saline. However, the optimal intravenous solution (isotonic saline, one-half isotonic saline, or isotonic sodium bicarbonate) and rate and duration of infusion remain unclear. In an uncontrolled prospective observational study reported 35 years ago, 100 consecutive patients undergoing angiography, of whom 25% had CKD (blood urea nitrogen > 30 mg/dL or serum creatinine >1.8 mg/dL), received 550 mL/h of saline during the procedure (Eisenberg et al., 1980). No cases of acute renal failure (defined as an increase in blood urea nitrogen of 50% or 20 mg/dL or a > 1-mg/dL increase in serum creatinine at 24 hours) were noted, despite the fact that up to 500 mL of contrast was administered. Although flawed in many respects, this study suggested that aggressive fluid administration may prevent or at least reduce the severity of contrast nephropathy. In the Nephrotoxic Effects in High-Risk Patients Undergoing Angiography (NEPHRIC) study comparing iohexol to iodixanol (Aspelin et al., 2003), it was recommended (but not required) that patients receive 500 mL of intravenous saline before angiography followed by 1 L of saline from the start of the procedure. Most controlled trials, however, have administered lesser amounts of fluids. In one study, isotonic (0.9%) saline was superior to half isotonic (0.45%) saline; this benefit was especially noted in diabetic patients and those given more than 250 mL of contrast (Weisbord and Palevsky, 2008). Some studies have suggested that isotonic bicarbonate may offer advantages over isotonic saline, presumably because of an antioxidant effect. Whether isotonic bicarbonate is superior to isotonic saline remains unclear, however, and is the subject of an ongoing large Veterans Affairs (VA) Cooperative Trial.

A popular regimen is to administer a bolus of 3 mL/kg of isotonic saline or bicarbonate for 1 hour prior to the procedure and continue the infusion at a rate of 1 mL/kg/h for 6 hours after the procedure. One issue with isotonic bicarbonate solution is that it requires compounding in the pharmacy. Moreover, bicarbonate administration carries the risk of worsening hypokalemia or further lowering of ionized calcium leading to symptomatic hypocalcemia in patients at risk of these complications (see Chapter 11). Until more conclusive evidence is forthcoming, many clinicians prefer to use isotonic saline rather than isotonic bicarbonate for prophylaxis.

Many pharmaceutical agents have been tried in an attempt to prevent radiocontrast nephropathy, the most studied being NAC (Mucomyst).

Others include theophylline, dopamine, fenoldopam, sodium citrate, atrial natriuretic peptide, ascorbic acid, trimethazine, nifedipine, captopril, and prostaglandins. None of these have proven value. Statins have also been evaluated, with potentially promising results. In one study, 2,998 patients with type 2 diabetes and stage 2 to 3 CKD were assigned to receive rosuvastatin (10 mg daily 2 days prior and 3 days after the scheduled procedure) or to a control group prior to a diagnostic angiogram with or without percutaneous intervention (Han et al., 2014). Contrast-induced AKI (defined as $\geq$0.5 mg/dL or $\geq$25% increase in serum creatinine above baseline at 72 hours after contrast exposure) was less common among patients assigned to rosuvastatin, compared with control (2.3% vs. 3.9%, respectively). The preventive effect of statins appears to be dose-related (Ukaigwe et al., 2014).

There are no data to suggest that performance of hemodialysis or hemofiltration to remove contrast has clinical benefits, either to prevent nephrotoxicity or to prevent other complications (Rodby, 2007).

USE OF CONTRAST-ENHANCED MRI

Most MRI contrast agents in clinical use are chelates of gadolinium. These agents can accumulate with renal failure since they are excreted in the urine. There are two major concerns with gadolinium: the possible development of NSF in patients with severe CKD; and the risk of nephrotoxicity, which has been suggested to be similar to that seen with iodinated contrast agents, especially when higher doses of gadolinium are employed.

Almost all cases of NSF that have been reported have been associated with gadolinium use, and most of these have been in patients on dialysis or with advanced renal failure (eGFR <30 mL/min/1.73 m^2) (Chrysochou et al., 2010). Patients with AKI are also presumably at high risk, as eGFR overestimates true GFR in such patients, which is virtually always less than 30 mL/min. The risk of NSF after gadolinium administration has not been defined in patients with lesser severity of CKD (eGFR between 30 and 60 mL/min/1.73 m^2). The decision to administer gadolinium in such patients needs to be individualized, as there are no data to estimate risk and no consensus among experts. Current guidelines state that gadolinium should be avoided if at all possible, when eGFR is less than 30 mL/min/1.73 m^2. If it must be given, Kidney Disease: Improving Global Outcomes (KDIGO, 2012) guidelines suggest use of macrocyclic chelate preparations (such as gadoteridol, gadobutrol, or gadoterate) and use of the lowest possible dose. Hemodialysis after the procedure to remove the contrast material should be considered. In patients with an eGFR in the 15- to 30-mL/min/1.73 m^2 range (stage 4 CKD), most would not perform hemodialysis after gadolinium administration unless there is an access already in place. However, in patients with an eGFR less than 15 mL/min/1.73 m^2 (stage 5 CKD) but not on dialysis and without vascular access, many nephrologists would place a temporary access and perform hemodialysis. In maintenance hemodialysis patients, hemodialysis should be performed as soon as possible after the imaging study. A second dialysis session at 24 hours should also be considered. Since clearance of gadolinium with peritoneal dialysis is low, such patients should receive hemodialysis to remove gadolinium or, if hemodialysis is not possible, rapid peritoneal exchanges.

Gadolinium-based contrast media are also associated with nephrotoxicity when given at high doses (>0.3 mmol/kg) for digital subtraction angiography. In one study, 21 patients with moderate to severe CKD (average serum creatinine concentration of 3.2 mg/dL [283 μmol/L]) undergoing digital subtraction angiography were randomly assigned to iodinated nonionic contrast media (iohexol) or gadolinium (gadobutrol) (Erley et al., 2004). The incidence of nephrotoxicity was similar and substantial (~50%) in both groups.

WHAT IS THE OPTIMAL APPROACH?

The most important consideration is to determine if the patient is at increased risk of radiocontrast nephropathy. The major risk factor is CKD, particularly in those with diabetes. In such patients, the best approach is to use alternative nontoxic imaging, such as ultrasonography, MRI without gadolinium contrast (such as time-of-flight MRI), or CT without contrast. If radiocontrast is needed, it is best to use the iso-osmotic agent iodixanol or nonionic low-osmolal agents such as iopamidol or ioversol rather than iohexol. The lowest possible dose should be employed, and repetitive studies within a short time period (<48 hours) should be avoided. Intravenous hydration should be given; one such regimen is 3 mL/kg of isotonic saline for 1 hour prior to the procedure, followed by 1 mL/kg/h for 6 hours after the procedure. There are no data to support hemodialysis or hemofiltration to remove radiocontrast, even in patients with severe CKD but not yet on dialysis. With respect to gadolinium, if it is utilized in patients on maintenance hemodialysis, dialysis treatment should be performed as soon as possible after its administration. This probably also applies to patients with stage 5 CKD (eGFR <15 mL/min/1.73 m^2) but not on dialysis.

An important caveat when considering gadolinium use in patients with severe CKD (eGFR <30 mL/min/m^2) or ESRD (end-stage renal disease) is that there is currently no evidence that removal of gadolinium actually decreases the risk of NSF. Therefore, the best option remains to avoid its use. If a contrast-enhanced study is essential in such patients, most clinicians believe that the use of the lowest possible dose of radiocontrast is preferred to administering gadolinium.

PATIENT 1

A 76-year-old man with a long history of diabetes mellitus and diabetic kidney disease with an eGFR of 25 mL/min/1.73 m^2 is admitted for pulmonary edema. He is given diuretics with clinical improvement. Blood pressure (BP) is 120/80 mm Hg and he is not anemic. It is determined by the cardiology service that the patient needs to undergo urgent coronary angiography and will require 100 to 200 mL of radiocontrast. A nephrologist is consulted to give an estimate of his risk for developing radiocontrast nephropathy severe enough to require dialysis.

Q: What is the risk in this situation?

A: This patient is clearly at substantial risk due to older age, severe diabetic kidney disease, and congestive heart failure. A number of online risk calculators are now available. Using one such calculator (Mehran et al., 2004), in which contrast-induced nephropathy is defined as an increase in serum creatinine of more than 25% or more than 0.5 mg/dL (44 µmol/L) from baseline within 48 hours after angiography, the risk of nephrotoxicity in this patient is 57% with a 12.6% risk of requiring dialysis.

PATIENT 2

A 40-year-old woman with autosomal dominant polycystic kidney disease is admitted to the hospital with headache and visual changes. She has severe CKD with an eGFR of 15 mL/min/1.73 m^2. She is mildly hypertensive (BP 150/90 mm Hg) not anemic. She does not have a dialysis access. A neurologist is concerned that she may have a cerebral aneurysm and wishes to obtain an MRI with contrast of the brain. A nephrologist is consulted and asked to perform hemodialysis to remove gadolinium immediately following the procedure.

Q: Is this the best approach?

A: This patient is at risk of developing NSF from administration of gadolinium. If it is absolutely necessary to administer gadolinium, many nephrologists would place a temporary hemodialysis catheter to perform hemodialysis as soon as possible after the end of the procedure. However, there is currently no evidence that dialysis will actually decrease the risk of NSF. A time-of-flight MRI without gadolinium would be a better option. Another approach would be to perform a CT with contrast, or if the clinical suspicion is very high, proceed directly to cerebral angiography. The risk of radiocontrast-induced nephropathy in this patient is calculated to be only about 15% but with less than a 1% chance of requiring dialysis.

References

Agmon Y, Peleg H, Greenfeld Z, et al. Nitric oxide and prostanoids protect the renal outer medulla from radiocontrast toxicity in the rat. *J Clin Invest*. 1994;94:1069.

Asif A, Epstein M. Prevention of radiocontrast-induced nephropathy. *Am J Kidney Dis*. 2004;44: 12–24.

Aspelin P, Aubry P, Fransson SG, et al. Nephrotoxic effects in high-risk patients undergoing angiography. *N Engl J Med*. 2003;348:491–499.

Chrysochou C, Power A, Shurrab AE, et al. Low risk for nephrogenic systemic fibrosis in nondialysis patients who have chronic kidney disease and are investigated with gadolinium-enhanced magnetic resonance imaging. *Clin J Am Soc Nephrol*. 2010;5:484–489.

Cigarroa RG, Lange RA, Williams RH, et al. Dosing of contrast material to prevent contrast nephropathy in patients with renal disease. *Am J Med*. 1989;86:649–652.

Eisenberg RL, Bank WO, Hedgcock MW. Renal failure after major angiography. *Am J Med*. 1980;68(1):43–46.

Erley CM, Bader BD, Berger ED, et al. Gadolinium-based contrast media compared with iodinated media for digital subtraction angiography in azotaemic patients. *Nephrol Dial Transplant*. 2004;19:2526–2531.

Han Y, Zhu G, Han L, et al. Short-term rosuvastatin therapy for prevention of contrast-induced acute kidney injury in patients with diabetes and chronic kidney disease. *J Am Coll Cardiol*. 2014;63:62–70.

Heyman SN, Rosenberger C, Rosen S. Regional alterations in renal haemodynamics and oxygenation: a role in contrast medium-induced nephropathy. *Nephrol Dial Transplant*. 2005;20(suppl 1):i6.

Kian K, Wyatt C, Schon D, et al. Safety of low-dose radiocontrast for interventional AV fistula salvage in stage 4 chronic kidney disease patients. *Kidney Int*. 2006;69:1444–1449.

Kidney Disease: Improving Global Outcomes. KDIGO clinical practice guideline for acute kidney injury. *Kidney Int*. 2012;2(suppl 1):69–88.

Kushner FG, Hand M, Smith SC Jr, et al. 2009 focused updates: ACC/AHA guidelines for the management of patients with ST-elevation myocardial infarction (updating the 2004 guideline and 2007 focused update) and ACC/AHA/SCAI guidelines on percutaneous coronary intervention (updating the 2005 guideline and 2007 focused update): a report of the American College of Cardiology Foundation/American Heart Association Task Force on Practice Guidelines. *J Am Coll Cardiol*. 2009;54:2205–2241.

Laskey W, Aspelin P, Davidson C, et al. Nephrotoxicity of iodixanol versus iopamidol in patients with chronic kidney disease and diabetes mellitus undergoing coronary angiographic procedures. *Am Heart J*. 2009;158:822–828.

Marenzi G, Assanelli E, Campodonico J, et al. Contrast volume during primary percutaneous coronary intervention and subsequent contrast-induced nephropathy and mortality. *Ann Intern Med*. 2009;150:170–177.

Mehran R, Aymong ED, Nikolsky E, et al. A simple risk score for prediction of contrast-induced nephropathy after percutaneous coronary intervention: development and initial validation. *J Am Coll Cardiol*. 2004;44(7):1393–1399.

Mendoza FA, Artlett CM, Sandorfi N, et al. Description of 12 cases of nephrogenic fibrosing dermopathy and review of the literature. *Semin Arthritis Rheum.* 2006;35:238–249.

Mitchell AM, Jones AE, Tumlin JA, et al. Incidence of contrast-induced nephropathy after contrast-enhanced computed tomography in the outpatient setting. *Clin J Am Soc Nephrol.* 2010;5:4.

Pannu N, Wiebe N, Tonelli M; Alberta Kidney Disease Network. Prophylaxis strategies for contrast-induced nephropathy. *JAMA.* 2006;295:2765–2779.

Parfrey PS, Griffiths SM, Barrett BJ, et al. Contrast material-induced renal failure in patients with diabetes mellitus, renal insufficiency, or both. A prospective controlled study. *N Engl J Med.* 1989;320:143.

Persson PB, Hansell P, Liss P. Pathophysiology of contrast medium-induced nephropathy. *Kidney Int.* 2005;68:14.

Reed M, Meier P, Tamhane UU, et al. The relative renal safety of iodixanol compared with low-osmolar contrast media: a meta-analysis of randomized controlled trials. *JACC Cardiovasc Interv.* 2009;2:645–654.

Rodby RA. Preventing complications of radiographic contrast media: is there a role for dialysis? *Semin Dial.* 2007;20(1):19–23.

Rudnick MR, Berns JS, Cohen RM, et al. Nephrotoxic risks of renal angiography: contrast media-associated nephrotoxicity and atheroembolism—a critical review. *Am J Kidney Dis.* 1994;24:713.

Rudnick MR, Davidson C, Laskey W, et al. Nephrotoxicity of iodixanol versus ioversol in patients with chronic kidney disease: the Visipaque Angiography/Interventions with Laboratory Outcomes in Renal Insufficiency (VALOR) Trial. *Am Heart J.* 2008;156:776–782.

Rudnick MR, Goldfarb S, Wexler L, et al. Nephrotoxicity of ionic and nonionic contrast media in 1196 patients: a randomized trial. The Iohexol Cooperative Study. *Kidney Int.* 1995;47:254–261.

Solomon RJ, Natarajan MK, Doucet S, et al. Cardiac Angiography in Renally Impaired Patients (CARE) study: a randomized double-blind trial of contrast-induced nephropathy in patients with chronic kidney disease. *Circulation.* 2007;115:3189–3196.

Stolker JM, McCullough PA, Rao S, et al. Pre-procedural glucose levels and the risk for contrast-induced acute kidney injury in patients undergoing coronary angiography. *J Am Coll Cardiol.* 2010;55:1433.

Ukaigwe A, Karmacharya P, Mahmood M, et al. Meta-analysis on efficacy of statins for prevention of contrast-induced acute kidney injury in patients undergoing coronary angiography. *Am J Cardiol.* 2014;114:1295–1302.

Weisbord SD, Mor MK, Resnick AL, et al. Incidence and outcomes of contrast-induced AKI following computed tomography. *Clin J Am Soc Nephrol.* 2008;3:1274.

Weisbord SD, Palevsky PM. Prevention of contrast-induced nephropathy with volume expansion. *Clin J Am Soc Nephrol.* 2008;3:273–280.

Is There a Risk to Rapidly Lowering the Plasma Potassium in Patients with Hyperkalemia?

15

Hyperkalemia is one of the most common and serious metabolic complications in patients with chronic kidney disease (CKD) and, in particular, end-stage renal disease (ESRD). Emergent treatment of hyperkalemia by administration of calcium to decrease cardiac repolarization and insulin to shift of potassium into cells is now standard and universally accepted. In most situations, potassium also needs to be removed from the body, either by diuretics, potassium-binding agents, or dialysis. These methods are generally quite effective in lowering plasma potassium levels and may be lifesaving as severe hyperkalemia can cause sudden cardiac death. But, is there also a risk of sudden cardiac death if the plasma potassium is lowered too quickly?

Several factors come into play when making a decision about how and how rapidly to lower plasma potassium in patients with hyperkalemia. First, the etiology of hyperkalemia needs to be considered. Potassium is the most prevalent cation in the body (total body potassium is ~50 mmol/kg), and most of it is in the intracellular fluid (ICF), with extracellular fluid (ECF) content normally only about 4 mmol/L $\times$ 17 L = 67 mmol. Disorders of potassium concentration can be due to an imbalance between intake and output of potassium (external potassium balance), an imbalance in distribution between the ECF and ICF (internal potassium balance), or both (Fig. 15.1). The plasma potassium concentration thus depends on total body potassium as well as its distribution between ECF and ICF. Certain conditions increase the ECF:ICF potassium ratio, leading to hyperkalemia without a change in total body potassium. More

Internal potassium balance   **External potassium balance**

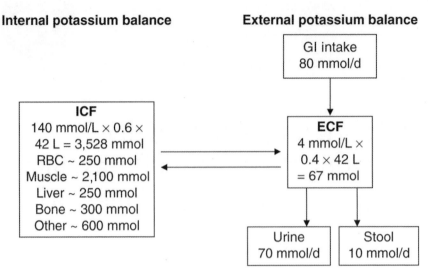

FIGURE 15.1 Internal and external potassium balance. The figure depicts typical potassium balance in a 70-kg man with a total body water of 42 L. (From Moinuddin IK, Leehey DJ. *Handbook of Nephrology*. Philadelphia, PA: Lippincott Williams & Wilkins; 2013.)

commonly, total body potassium is also increased. If the problem is increased ECF:ICF ratio with normal total body potassium, shifting potassium back into cells may be the only therapy needed (e.g., administration of insulin in hyperglycemic patients). On the other hand, if total body potassium is increased, potassium will need to be removed from the body. Table 15.1 lists common causes of hyperkalemia.

The urgency of treatment of hyperkalemia depends upon its acuity and whether or not there are symptoms and signs attributable to hyperkalemia (EKG changes and/or muscle weakness). One situation in which overly aggressive treatment of hyperkalemia can result in potentially catastrophic results is uncontrolled diabetes, in particular diabetic ketoacidosis. In these patients, lack of insulin leads to decreased cellular potassium uptake, resulting in hyperkalemia even though the total body potassium is often reduced (due to osmotic diuresis from hyperglycemia, poor dietary intake, and gastrointestinal (GI) losses). The increased ECF:ICF ratio in such patients is rapidly reversed by the administration of insulin. Because of whole-body potassium deficiency, hypokalemia frequently ensues during subsequent therapy, and failure to administer adequate potassium can lead to hypokalemia and potentially fatal complications. At the other end of the spectrum, in hyperkalemic patients with marked tissue breakdown (e.g., rhabdomyolysis, hemolysis, tumor

Etiologies of Hyperkalemia

Normal Total Body Potassium (Increased ECF:ICF Ratio)
Metabolic acidosis (inorganic)
Insulin deficiency
Drugs (digoxin, beta-blockers)
Acute hypertonicity (osmolar water and K shift out of cells)
Hyperkalemic periodic paralysis (very rare)

High Total Body Potassium (Decreased Excretion with or without Increased Exogenous Intake)
Acute or chronic kidney disease
Medications that impair potassium excretion
  Potassium-sparing diuretics
  Renin–angiotensin system (RAS) inhibitors
  Heparin (inhibits biosynthesis of aldosterone)
  Nonsteroidal anti-inflammatory drugs (NSAIDs)
  Calcineurin inhibitors
  Trimethoprim
Adrenal insufficiency
Selective hypoaldosteronism
Hyperkalemic renal tubular acidosis
Salt substitutes (in patients with kidney disease)

High Total Body Potassium (Increased ECF:ICF Ratio Coupled with Decreased Excretion)
Cell breakdown (hemolysis, rhabdomyolysis, tumor lysis, shock)

---

lysis syndrome, shock), release of potassium from damaged cells can raise plasma levels rapidly; such patients generally require urgent therapy.

INSULIN/GLUCOSE

It has now been known for a quarter century that in a normoglycemic patient, the "standard therapy" of 10 units of intravenous regular insulin followed immediately by 50 mL (one "amp") of 50% glucose (25 g) can result in the development of hypoglycemia in up to 75% of patients (Allon and Copkney, 1990). However, many sources still recommend this regimen (i.e., insulin:dextrose 1 unit:2.5 g). Administration of 10 units of regular insulin with 100 mL (two "amps" or 50 g of glucose, i.e., insulin:dextrose 1 unit:5 g) is a safer alternative. The effect of regular insulin begins in 10 to 20 minutes, peaks at 30 to 60 minutes, and lasts for 4 to 6 hours. Therefore, late hypoglycemia can occasionally occur, leading some to recommend an infusion of 10% glucose for 4 to 6 hours after the initial bolus, though this is not common practice. The plasma potassium concentration will typically decrease by 0.5 to 1.5 mmol/L with this therapy.

ALBUTEROL

Since activation of the beta-2-receptor also shifts potassium into cells, beta-2-adrenergic agonists such as albuterol can be effective in the acute treatment of hyperkalemia. However, the dose that has been studied is 10 to 20 mg in 4 mL of saline by nebulization over 10 minutes (which is four to eight times the dose used for bronchodilation), which can have cardiac side effects. Insulin and albuterol have additive effects, with the combination reducing plasma potassium concentration by about 1.5 mmol/L (Allon and Copkney, 1990).

SODIUM BICARBONATE

Sodium bicarbonate traditionally was part of the standard cocktail (calcium, insulin/glucose, bicarbonate) used to treat hyperkalemia. Increasing systemic pH leads to hydrogen ion shift out of cells in exchange for potassium shift into cells. Moreover, bicarbonate administration has been shown to shift potassium into cells by a pH-independent mechanism (Fraley and Adler, 1977). However, the effect of bicarbonate is not always predictable, and indeed, may have no effect in hemodialysis patients (Blumberg et al., 1988). It is probably best reserved for nonhemodialysis patients with concomitant metabolic acidosis. In some circumstances, for instance, a patient presenting with severe hyperkalemia, hyperchloremic metabolic acidosis, and volume depletion, administration of isotonic sodium bicarbonate (i.e., 150 mmol in 1 L of 5% dextrose in water) will effectively treat all three conditions.

In all urgent situations, calcium and insulin and sometimes bicarbonate should be given to protect the heart and shift potassium into cells. These effects will only be transient however, and in most cases, additional therapy to remove potassium from the body will be required. This can be accomplished by diuretics, potassium-binding agents, or dialysis.

Dialysis is indicated if other measures are ineffective, hyperkalemia is severe or is expected to worsen, or there are other coexisting reasons to perform dialysis. Hemodialysis can remove 25 to 50 mmol of potassium per hour (Ahmed and Weisberg, 2001). One of the major determinants of the rate of potassium removal is the potassium gradient between the plasma and dialysate. One must also keep in mind postdialysis potassium rebound, which occurs because of movement of potassium out of cells into the plasma for several hours after cessation of dialysis. This generally results in about a 1-mmol/L increase in plasma potassium within 4 hours of the termination of dialysis, with most of the increase occurring in the first 90 minutes postdialysis (Blumberg et al., 1997). For this reason, measurement of immediate postdialysis plasma potassium concentration should generally be avoided, since the results are likely to be misleading and may lead to inappropriate potassium therapy. Peritoneal dialysis and continuous therapies are much less effective than hemodialysis in removing potassium.

What dialysate potassium concentration should be employed? There are few more controversial areas in nephrology. Many nephrologists have been trained using the "rule of 8s," that is, the sum of the patient's plasma potassium and the dialysate potassium level should equal 8. Although a practical guideline, especially in the outpatient setting, this has never been tested in a clinical trial. Moreover, its use will result in rapid lowering of plasma potassium concentration in patients with hyperkalemia (e.g., a patient with a plasma potassium of 7 mmol/L would be dialyzed with a dialysate potassium of 1 mmol/L according to this formulation), which may have deleterious consequences as discussed in the following.

The typical potassium concentration in the dialysate for acute hemodialysis ranges from 2 to 4 mmol/L and depends on the predialysis plasma potassium concentration. There is no general consensus concerning the optimal strategy in hyperkalemic patients. The following is one approach:

Plasma potassium less than 4 mmol/L: Use a dialysate potassium concentration of 4 mmol/L to prevent the development of hypokalemia and its complications.

Plasma potassium between 4 and 5.5 mmol/L: A dialysate potassium concentration in the 3- to 4-mmol/L range is appropriate. If a rapid increase in extracellular potassium is anticipated prior to the next hemodialysis session (e.g., due to marked rhabdomyolysis), then a dialysate potassium of 2 mmol/L to ensure normokalemia may obviate the need for daily dialysis for hyperkalemia. However, caution is advised in patients who are at risk for arrhythmias related to potassium removal (such as those with coronary artery disease, left ventricular hypertrophy [LVH], digoxin use, hypertension, and advanced age), and some would avoid using a dialysate potassium less than 3 mmol/L. This is because the potassium concentration gradient across the cell membrane is critical for the repolarization process, and large potassium fluxes during dialysis may lead to inhomogeneous repolarization allowing for the onset of re-entrant arrhythmias. In such patients, frequent and complex arrhythmias can develop during hemodialysis sessions when a dialysate potassium of 2 mmol/L is employed (Morrison et al., 1980).

Plasma potassium between 5.5 and 8 mmol/L: A 2 mmol/L dialysate potassium bath is generally used, with the above caveat that some would not use a dialysate potassium less than 3 mmol/L.

Plasma potassium more than 8 mmol/L: This is the most controversial area. Some will use a dialysate potassium concentration of 1 mmol/L (or even potassium-free dialysate if the situation is deemed life-threatening). The effects of very low potassium dialysates in such patients have not been well studied. In one study of 11 stable hemodialysis patients with no history of arrhythmia or digitalis use, in which dialysates with potassium concentrations of 2, 1, or 0 mmol/L were compared in a crossover fashion, the potassium-free dialysate removed significantly more potassium (78.5 ± 2.6 mmol) than the 1-K dialysate (62.9 ± 5.1 mmol) or the 2-K dialysate (50.6 ± 6 mmol) (Hou et al., 1989). Only one patient had high-grade ventricular ectopy, which was seen with each of the three potassium concentrations, but was most severe with the potassium-free dialysate. From this study, it is clear that low or zero potassium dialysate is more effective in removing potassium, but the small sample size, exclusion of patients with a history of cardiac arrhythmias, and the absence of predialysis hyperkalemia make it impossible to apply these observations to the management of severely hyperkalemic patients who may have underlying cardiac disease. To minimize the risk of arrhythmia, some proponents of 0 or 1 mmol/L dialysates will check the plasma potassium every 30 to 60 minutes during dialysis, and once the plasma potassium is between 6 and 7 mmol/L, increase the dialysate potassium concentration to 2 mmol/L for the remainder of the treatment. There are no data to support this approach.

A better approach to treat severe hyperkalemia in hemodialysis patients may be to "ramp down" the dialysate potassium so that the gradient between the plasma and dialysate is minimized. One prospective, multicenter, randomized crossover study of 42 patients examined the incidence of ventricular arrhythmias with two different dialysate potassium concentration protocols (Redaelli et al., 1996). One arm of the study was designed to maintain a constant plasma-to-dialysate potassium concentration gradient throughout the dialysis procedure, while the other arm consisted of the standard constant dialysate potassium concentration, which results in a varying potassium gradient. Treatment with the constant plasma-to-dialysate potassium gradient protocol resulted in 36% and 32% reductions in rate of premature ventricular contractions and ventricular couplets during hemodialysis, respectively, compared with dialysis using a constant dialysate potassium concentration. Another crossover study (Muñoz et al., 2008) compared potassium-profiled hemodialysis to constant potassium hemodialysis in 12 elderly patients with cardiac arrhythmias or at a high risk for arrhythmia (advanced age, hypertension, LVH, heart valve disease, coronary artery disease, diabetes, paroxysmal atrial fibrillation). In the potassium-profiled group, the potassium concentration in the dialysate was high (3.2–4 mmol/L) at the beginning of treatment and was progressively reduced throughout the dialysis session to 1 to 1.3 mmol/L. The mean dialysate potassium concentration was 2 mmol/L in both groups. There was a significant reduction of postdialysis corrected QT interval in the profiled group compared with the constant potassium group. Moreover, the severity and mean number of ventricular extrasystoles also decreased in the profiled group. Finally, in a study of 30 arrhythmia-prone hemodialysis patients, use of a constant (2.5 mmol/L) potassium dialysate was compared to decreasing dialysate potassium protocol (Santoro et al., 2008). Overall, there was no difference in arrhythmias between the groups, but in a subset of patients prone to developing arrhythmia during dialysis, the decreasing potassium protocol was less arrhythmogenic than the constant potassium protocol. However, the effect was greatest many hours after the end of dialysis, casting some doubt on whether potassium gradient during the treatment was causing the arrhythmias.

Whether avoiding very low dialysate potassium will prevent sudden deaths should be tested in adequately powered clinical trials. It is unfortunate that, in view of the importance of this common problem, such a clinical trial has not yet been done. In the absence of a large randomized clinical trial, the author favors a modified "ramped" approach (or "stepped" approach) for the treatment of severe hyperkalemia (plasma potassium >7 mmol/L), with use of an initial dialysate potassium concentration of 3 to 4 mmol/L with a reduction to 2 to 3 mmol/L for the second half of the treatment. In the opinion of the author, dialysate potassium concentrations less than 2 mmol/L should be avoided in all patients.

PATIENT 1

A 65-year-old woman is undergoing rehabilitation at the local hospital. She has a long history of hypertension, diabetes, and CKD, with an eGFR of 20 mL/min/1.73 m^2. Medications include insulin, furosemide, enalapril, and potassium supplements. A nephrologist is called to see her for severe hyperkalemia (plasma potassium of 6.8 mmol/L) accompanied by hyperglycemia (blood glucose of 500 mg/dL). The plasma potassium done 1 week previously was 5 mmol/L. A stat EKG is ordered, which reveals peaked T waves. The patient is asymptomatic. The nurse states that the patient was at x-ray that morning and did not receive her usual daily insulin dose.

Q: What is the best approach?

1. Administer a potassium-binding agent
2. Administer insulin
3. Discontinue enalapril and potassium supplements
4. Perform emergency hemodialysis
5. All of the above except (4)

A: This patient has chronic hyperkalemia from CKD in conjunction with administration of angiotensin-converting-enzyme (ACE) inhibitor and potassium supplements. The severe hyperkalemia was precipitated by failure to give insulin. Thus, it is predicted that both total body potassium and ECF:ICF ratio are elevated. Shifting potassium into cells with insulin in combination with administration of a potassium-binding agent to remove potassium from the body is the best approach. Since the patient is very hyperglycemic, 10 units of regular insulin without dextrose should be administered intravenously. Enalapril and potassium should also be discontinued. There is no indication for emergency hemodialysis unless the plasma potassium cannot be lowered by the aforementioned interventions.

PATIENT 2

A 78-year-old man with ESRD on maintenance dialysis is admitted to the hospital with weakness. He has hypertension, LVH, coronary artery disease, and diabetes. On examination, he is comfortable and euvolemic but has decreased muscle strength throughout. The plasma potassium concentration is 8.5 mmol/L. An EKG shows peaked T waves and prolongation of the PR interval with flattening of the P waves. After administration of intravenous calcium gluconate and insulin coupled with dextrose, urgent hemodialysis is performed.

Q: What is the best initial dialysis prescription?

1. 0 K
2. 1 mmol/L K
3. 2 mmol/L K
4. 3 mmol/L K

A: As indicated in the text, this is a very controversial area of nephrology. An important consideration is that any of the aforementioned prescriptions will lower plasma potassium. The safest approach is to initially use a 3 mmol/L K dialysate, as use of lower potassium dialysate will lead to a more rapid decrease in plasma potassium and increase the risk of arrhythmia in this elderly patient with heart disease. The plasma potassium should be repeated after 1 to 2 hours of dialysis. If the plasma potassium is still more than 6 mmol/L, changing to a 2-mmol/L K dialysate is reasonable for the remainder of dialysis. Another option would be to continue using the 3-mmol/L K dialysate but extend the duration of dialysis from the usual 4 hours to 5 to 6 hours, though this is uncommonly done in practice.

References

Ahmed J, Weisberg LS. Hyperkalemia in dialysis patients. *Semin Dial.* 2001;14:348–356.

Allon M, Copkney C. Albuterol and insulin for treatment of hyperkalemia in hemodialysis patients. *Kidney Int.* 1990;38:869–872.

Blumberg A, Roser HW, Zehnder C, et al. Plasma potassium in patients with terminal renal failure during and after haemodialysis: relationship with dialytic potassium removal and total body potassium. *Nephrol Dial Transplant.* 1997;12:1629–1634.

Blumberg A, Weidmann P, Shaw S, et al. Effect of various therapeutic approaches on plasma potassium and major regulating factors in terminal renal failure. *Am J Med.* 1988;85:507–512.

Fraley DS, Adler S. Correction of hyperkalemia by bicarbonate despite constant blood pH. *Kidney Int.* 1977;12:354–360.

Hou S, McElroy PA, Nootens J, et al. Safety and efficacy of low-potassium dialysate. *Am J Kidney Dis.* 1989;13:137–143.

Morrison G, Michelson EL, Brown S, et al. Mechanism and prevention of cardiac arrhythmias in chronic hemodialysis patients. *Kidney Int.* 1980;17(6):811–819.

Muñoz RI, Montenegro J, Salcedo A, et al. Effect of acetate-free biofiltration with a potassium-profiled dialysate on the control of cardiac arrhythmias in patients at risk: a pilot study. *Hemodial Int.* 2008;12(1):108–113.

Redaelli B, Locatelli F, Limido D, et al. Effect of a new model of hemodialysis potassium removal on the control of ventricular arrhythmias. *Kidney Int.* 1996;50:609–617.

Santoro A, Mancini E, London G, et al. Patients with complex arrhythmias during and after haemodialysis suffer from different regimens of potassium removal. *Nephrol Dial Transplant.* 2008;23(4):1415–1421.

16

Should Calcium-Based Phosphate Binders Be Used in Patients with Chronic Kidney Disease?

Phosphate retention develops early in chronic kidney disease (CKD) due to the reduction in the glomerular filtration rate (GFR) and filtered phosphate load (Slatopolsky et al., 1968). An increase in phosphaturic hormones such as parathyroid hormone (PTH) and fibroblast growth factor 23 (FGF-23) help to maintain phosphate balance, but eventually overt hyperphosphatemia develops, usually when the GFR is less than 30 mL/min/1.73 m². Uncontrolled hyperphosphatemia is a major risk factor for what is now termed chronic kidney disease–metabolic bone disease (CKD-MBD) (Stevens et al., 2004; Young et al., 2004). Most patients with hyperphosphatemia are currently treated with phosphate binders, but there is a paucity of high-grade evidence supporting their use.

NONDIALYSIS CKD

A large-scale clinical trial demonstrating the benefit of phosphate binders in nondialysis CKD is not available, and treatment recommendations are based on observational study findings and expert opinion (Kidney Disease: Improving Global Outcomes [KDIGO], 2009, 2013). Increased serum phosphorus has been associated with increased mortality among nondialysis CKD patients. In a meta-analysis of three studies with 4,651 such patients, there was a 35% increase in mortality per 1-mg/dL increase in serum phosphorus above normal (Palmer et al., 2011). Normalization of plasma phosphorus (i.e., <4.5 mg/dL [1.45 mmol/L]) is recommended by the KDIGO guidelines.

DIALYSIS PATIENTS

Increased serum phosphorus is also associated with increased mortality among dialysis patients (Block et al., 1998; Palmer et al., 2011). In a meta-analysis of 12 studies that included 92,345 patients with CKD, over 97% of whom were on dialysis (Palmer et al., 2011), serum phosphate of more than 5.5 mg/dL (1.78 mmol/L) was associated with increased mortality, with an 18% increase in risk for each 1-mg/dL increase in serum phosphorus. Maintaining the serum phosphorus concentration between 3.5 and 5.5 mg/dL (1.13 and 1.78 mmol/L) is recommended by the Kidney Disease Outcomes Quality Initiative (K/DOQI) guidelines (National Kidney Foundation, 2003). This, however, differs from the more recent KDIGO guidelines, which recommend lowering levels toward the normal range, but do not specify a specific target. As with nondialysis CKD, no randomized study has evaluated whether achieving these serum phosphate targets with phosphate binders affects clinically important outcomes in dialysis patients.

TREATMENT

Since the link between hyperphosphatemia and mortality has not been accompanied by data demonstrating that lowering serum phosphorus decreases mortality risk, it is important that any treatment for hyperphosphatemia should carry minimal risk itself. This issue will be examined in the following sections.

RESTRICTION OF PHOSPHORUS INTAKE

The treatment with the least risk is restriction of phosphate intake, providing it is done in a manner that does not result in limitation of nutritional intake. Phosphate restriction should therefore focus on avoidance of phosphate additives added to processed foods and drinks, and not high-biologic-value foods such as meat and eggs. The amount of phosphate additives in foods has doubled in the past 25 years, and this is likely the major reason for the continued high prevalence of hyperphosphatemia in end-stage renal disease (ESRD) patients despite improvements in dialysis therapy during this time. The phosphate in highly processed foods and drinks, which have high phosphate content, is not bound

TABLE 16.1	Phosphate Additives in Foods and Drinks

Processed meats and "enhanced" fresh meats
Chicken nuggets
Hot dogs
Luncheon meats
"Enhanced" fresh meats at many large grocery chain stores
Bottled drinks
Colas
Many other bottled drinks, including iced tea, lemonade, fruit drinks, fruit punch, and
    flavored waters
Avoid foods and drinks with word "phosphate" or "phosphoric acid" on the nutrition label
    Examples of phosphorus additives to avoid:
        Phosphoric acid (present in colas)
        Monosodium, disodium, or trisodium phosphate
        Sodium acid pyrophosphate
        Tetrasodium pyrophosphate
        Sodium or potassium tripolyphosphate
        Trisodium triphosphate
        Calcium phosphate

to phytates and is more easily absorbed compared with phosphate in fresh, unprocessed foods (Uribarri and Calvo, 2003). Patients must be instructed to read food labels and to identify phosphate-containing additives (Table 16.1). Limiting the intake of phosphate-containing food additives has been shown to be effective in reducing the serum phosphorus concentration in dialysis patients in a randomized trial (Sullivan et al., 2009).

PHOSPHATE BINDERS

Phosphate binders are categorized as calcium-containing and non–calcium-containing binders. Calcium-containing binders include calcium carbonate and calcium acetate. Non–calcium-containing binders include aluminum, sevelamer, and lanthanum. In the early days of maintenance dialysis, calcium carbonate was commonly used, but a not-infrequent problem was the development of hypercalcemia. Subsequently, aluminum-containing binders were in vogue, but it turned out that enough aluminum was absorbed to cause aluminum toxicity, which could be fatal, and calcium-containing binders, in particular calcium acetate, were again widely prescribed. More recently, there has been increased use of non–calcium-containing binders, in particular the cationic ion-exchange polymer sevelamer and the rare earth mineral lanthanum.

EFFECTS OF CALCIUM-CONTAINING BINDERS IN CKD PATIENTS

Because of impaired renal excretion of calcium, administration of calcium in CKD patients is expected to result in a positive calcium balance. A randomized, placebo-controlled crossover study examined the effect of oral calcium carbonate administration on calcium and phosphate balance in eight patients with stage 3 to 4 CKD (mean estimated GFR [eGFR] of 15–59 mL/min/1.73 m^2) (Hill et al., 2013). Subjects received a controlled diet with either a calcium carbonate supplement (1,500 mg/day calcium) or placebo and underwent two 3-week balance periods. Patients were in neutral calcium and phosphorus balance while on the placebo. Calcium carbonate supplementation had no effect on phosphorus balance, as decreased absorption was balanced by decreased urine phosphorus excretion. However, it caused a positive calcium balance; of note, the amount of calcium that was deposited in bone was less than the overall positive calcium balance, suggesting that some degree of soft-tissue deposition occurred. This study raises the question as to efficacy and safety of calcium-containing phosphate binders in nondialysis CKD patients.

In dialysis patients, use of large amounts of calcium-containing phosphate binders in the face of hyperphosphatemia has been shown to increase vascular calcification. In a seminal observation, 39 young dialysis patients and control subjects underwent electron beam computed tomography (EBCT) to detect coronary artery calcification (CAC) (Goodman et al., 2000). CAC was much more common in dialysis patients (88% vs. 5% in controls). Among the dialysis patients, the daily dose of calcium was twice as high in those with CAC as in those without CAC. This raised the possibility that calcium-containing phosphate binders might be causing CAC.

In order to address this possibility, in the Treat to Goal study, 200 patients undergoing maintenance hemodialysis were randomly assigned to sevelamer or calcium-containing phosphate binders (Chertow et al., 2002). After 12 months, although serum phosphorus control was similar with both agents, only calcium-based phosphate binders were associated with increased vascular calcification. In the subsequent RIND trial, 129 patients new to hemodialysis were randomly assigned to sevelamer or calcium-containing phosphate binders (Block et al., 2005). Among those with CAC at dialysis initiation, patients on sevelamer were more likely than those on calcium-containing phosphate binders to show stabilization or regression in CAC at 12 months. Neither study was powered to demonstrate a possible mortality benefit of sevelamer. Moreover, the interpretation of both studies is made more difficult by the fact that sevelamer has other potential beneficial effects in addition to phosphate lowering, including lipid lowering and reduction in inflammation and oxidative stress. In the subsequent CARE-2 trial, 203 hemodialysis patients with serum phosphorus levels more than 5.5 mg/dL, LDL-C levels more than 80 mg/dL, and CAC were randomly assigned to calcium acetate or to sevelamer for 12 months. Both groups received atorvastatin to obtain LDL-C levels less than 70 mg/dL. There was similar progression of CAC with sevelamer and calcium acetate (Qunibi et al., 2008). The conclusion of this trial was that, if lipids are lowered to a similar degree, there is no difference between calcium acetate and sevelamer on progression of CAC.

Among nondialysis CKD patients, sevelamer has also been associated with decreased vascular calcification compared to calcium. In the INDEPENDENT study, a randomized, multicenter, pilot study in stage 3 CKD (eGFR 30–60 mL/min/1.73 m^2), regression of vascular calcification at 12 months occurred in 24% of patients treated with sevelamer but in only 2% of those treated with calcium carbonate. By 24 months, new vascular calcification developed in only 5% of patients taking sevelamer versus 45% of those taking calcium carbonate (Di Iorio et al., 2012).

There are less data concerning lanthanum, but it also appears to be associated with less vascular calcification than calcium (Wada and Wada, 2014). In a randomized trial of 96 nondialysis CKD patients (eGFR 20–45 mL/min/1.73 m^2) in which lanthanum, sevelamer, calcium acetate, and placebo were all compared, calcium acetate appeared to cause a greater increase in vascular calcification than the other active treatments or placebo (Block et al., 2012).

PHOSPHATE BINDERS AND MORTALITY

Observational data support a mortality benefit of phosphate binders. In a prospective, observational study of 10,044 incident dialysis patients followed for 1 year, the use of phosphate binders was associated with a 25% lower 1-year mortality (Isakova et al., 2009). Among 6,797 patients enrolled in an observational, prospective study (COSMOS), patients prescribed phosphate binders had a 29% lower risk of all-cause mortality and a 22% lower risk of cardiovascular mortality (Cannata-Andía et al., 2013). Despite these epidemiological observations, randomized trials are needed to determine whether the use of phosphate binders decrease mortality or at least decrease clinically important endpoints in dialysis patients.

If one makes a "leap of faith" that phosphate binders are beneficial, which binder(s) should be employed? In view of evidence for calcium accumulation and vascular calcification associated with calcium-containing binders when compared to non–calcium binders, why are calcium-based binders so commonly used? One reason is cost, as they are less expensive than sevelamer and much less expensive than lanthanum. They are also favored by most clinicians for hypocalcemic patients, where an increase in serum calcium into the normal range will inhibit PTH levels and probably improve bone mineralization. Even in normocalcemic patients, most guidelines continue to recommend the use of calcium-containing phosphate binders in patients with no evidence of vascular calcification or adynamic bone disease. Such guidelines require clinical knowledge about these disorders, however, which is not always available or considered. Clearly, hypercalcemic patients should be treated with non–calcium-containing phosphate binders, especially if the cause of hypercalcemia (e.g., vitamin D, markedly elevated PTH) cannot be rectified.

One advantage of sevelamer is that due to its anion-binding effects, it also binds fatty acids and decreases LDL cholesterol, similar to the effect of cholestyramine or colestipol. As mentioned earlier, decreased CAC associated with this agent may be due to this lipid-lowering effect (Qunibi et al., 2008). The clinical benefit of lipid lowering in dialysis patients is controversial, as lowering cholesterol with statins has not been proven to be beneficial in such patients (Wanner et al., 2005; Fellström et al., 2009; Baigent et al., 2011). However, statins are beneficial in nondialysis CKD (Baigent et al., 2011), and such patients would be expected to benefit from the lipid-lowering effect of sevelamer. Another agent that may both lower phosphorus (by preventing intestinal absorption) and improve lipids is prolonged-release nicotinic acid (Niaspan), though more studies are needed.

Recently, a new option for managing hyperphosphatemia while simultaneously providing iron therapy became available. Ferric citrate hydrate has been shown to be effective in reducing serum phosphorus and FGF-23 concentrations while simultaneously increasing serum iron (Yokoyama et al., 2014). However, it must be kept in mind that citrate markedly enhances the absorption of aluminum, which can cause aluminum toxicity in patients taking aluminum-containing antacids (Bakir, 1989).

In summary, although a definitive statement is not possible, the use of calcium-containing binders in dialysis patients may not be advisable, as there are clear data that such therapy increases the risk of vascular calcification. Calcium-containing binders also appear to increase vascular calcification in nondialysis CKD patients. Since urinary calcium excretion is markedly decreased even in moderate CKD, it is expected that such patients will develop positive calcium balance with calcium-containing binders. On the basis of all the available data, the author prefers the use of non–calcium-containing binders such as sevelamer rather than calcium-containing phosphate binders in most nondialysis CKD and dialysis patients unless they are overtly hypocalcemic.

PATIENT 1

A 50-year-old woman with CKD due to polycystic kidney disease is seen in the renal clinic. Her plasma creatinine is 2 mg/dL with an eGFR of 30 mL/min/1.73 m². Her plasma calcium and phosphorus are 9 mg/dL (normal range 8.5–10 mg/dL) and 4.5 mg/dL (normal range 2.5–4.5 mg/dL), respectively, 25-hydroxy-vitamin D is 35 ng/mL (normal range 30–100 ng/mL), and her plasma intact PTH is 150 pg/mL (normal range 10–65 pg/mL).

Q: What would you recommend?

1. Phosphorus-restricted diet
2. Restriction of foods containing phosphate additives
3. Cholecalciferol (vitamin D_3) supplements
4. Calcitriol 0.25 µg thrice weekly to inhibit PTH

A: This patient has mild secondary hyperparathyroidism due to CKD. Phosphorus accumulation even in the absence of overt hyperphosphatemia can stimulate FGF-23 and PTH, which can ultimately lead to bone disease and mineral deposition in soft tissues. She is vitamin D_3 replete, so D_3 supplements are unlikely to be of benefit. A phosphorus-restricted diet carried out under the supervision of a trained dietitian is an option, but care must be taken to avoid malnutrition. The best approach is training the patient to avoid phosphate additives in foods. If this is not successful in lowering the PTH, administration of calcitriol is the next step, although evidence for benefit is not robust.

PATIENT 2

A 50-year-old man with ESRD due to diabetes mellitus on maintenance thrice weekly hemodialysis has routine monthly laboratories done. His plasma calcium and phosphorus are 9 mg/dL (normal range 8.5–10 mg/dL) and 6.5 mg/dL (normal range 2.5–4.5 mg/dL), respectively,

25-hydroxy-vitamin D is 35 ng/mL (normal range 30–100 ng/mL), and her plasma intact PTH is 450 pg/mL (normal range 10–65 pg/mL).

Q: What would you recommend?

1. Phosphorus-restricted diet
2. Restriction of foods containing phosphate additives
3. Calcitriol 0.25 µg thrice weekly to inhibit PTH
4. Calcium acetate 1,334 mg thrice daily with meals
5. Sevelamer carbonate 1,600 mg thrice daily with meals

A: This patient has moderate secondary hyperparathyroidism due to ESRD. Phosphorus restriction is clearly indicated in the presence of overt hyperphosphatemia. However, this is unlikely to normalize plasma phosphorus. Administration of calcitriol should decrease PTH, but since active vitamin D will increase intestinal absorption of both calcium and phosphorus, it may worsen hyperphosphatemia and raise the "calcium–phosphorus product." Phosphate binders are indicated. Calcium acetate is problematic in middle-aged patients with diabetes and ESRD who are very likely to have vascular calcification. Sevelamer will improve hyperphosphatemia without increasing calcium load and is probably the preferred therapy in this situation.

References

Baigent C, Landray MJ, Reith C, et al. The effects of lowering LDL cholesterol with simvastatin plus ezetimibe in patients with chronic kidney disease (Study of Heart and Renal Protection): a randomised placebo-controlled trial. *Lancet.* 2011;377:2181–2192.

Bakir AA. Acute aluminemic encephalopathy in chronic renal failure: the citrate factor. *Int J Artif Organs.* 1989;12(12):741–743.

Block GA, Hulbert-Shearon TE, Levin NW, et al. Association of serum phosphorus and calcium × phosphate product with mortality risk in chronic hemodialysis patients: a national study. *Am J Kidney Dis.* 1998;31:607–617.

Block GA, Spiegel DM, Ehrlich J, et al. Effects of sevelamer and calcium on coronary artery calcification in patients new to hemodialysis. *Kidney Int.* 2005;68:1815–1824.

Block GA, Wheeler DC, Persky MS, et al. Effects of phosphate binders in moderate CKD. *J Am Soc Nephrol.* 2012;23:1407–1415.

Cannata-Andía JB, Fernández-Martín JL, Locatelli F, et al. Use of phosphate-binding agents is associated with a lower risk of mortality. *Kidney Int.* 2013;84(5):998–1008.

Chertow GM, Burke SK, Raggi P; Treat to Goal Working Group. Sevelamer attenuates the progression of coronary and aortic calcification in hemodialysis patients. *Kidney Int.* 2002;62:245–252.

Di Iorio B, Bellasi A, Russo D; INDEPENDENT Study Investigators. Mortality in kidney disease patients treated with phosphate binders: a randomized study. *Clin J Am Soc Nephrol.* 2012;7:487–493.

Fellström BC, Jardine AG, Schmieder RE, et al. Rosuvastatin and cardiovascular events in patients undergoing hemodialysis. *N Engl J Med.* 2009;360:1395–1407.

Goodman WG, Goldin J, Kuizon BD, et al. Coronary-artery calcification in young adults with end-stage renal disease who are undergoing dialysis. *N Engl J Med*. 2000;342:1478–1483.

Hill KM, Martin BR, Wastney ME, et al. Oral calcium carbonate affects calcium but not phosphorus balance in stage 3-4 chronic kidney disease. *Kidney Int*. 2013;83:959–966.

Isakova T, Gutiérrez OM, Chang Y, et al. Phosphorus binders and survival on hemodialysis. *J Am Soc Nephrol*. 2009;20(2):388–396.

Kidney Disease: Improving Global Outcomes. KDIGO 2012 clinical practice guideline for the evaluation and management of chronic kidney disease. *Kidney Int Suppl*. 2013;3:5.

Kidney Disease: Improving Global Outcomes (KDIGO) CKD-MBD Work Group. KDIGO clinical practice guideline for the diagnosis, evaluation, prevention, and treatment of Chronic Kidney Disease–Mineral and Bone Disorder (CKD-MBD). *Kidney Int Suppl*. 2009;76(113):S1–S130.

National Kidney Foundation. K/DOQI clinical practice guidelines for bone metabolism and disease in chronic kidney disease. *Am J Kidney Dis*. 2003;42(4)(suppl 3):S1–S201.

Palmer SC, Hayen A, Macaskill P, et al. Serum levels of phosphorus, parathyroid hormone, and calcium and risks of death and cardiovascular disease in individuals with chronic kidney disease: a systematic review and meta-analysis. *JAMA*. 2011;305:1119–1127.

Qunibi W, Moustafa M, Muenz LR, et al. A 1-year randomized trial of calcium acetate versus sevelamer on progression of coronary artery calcification in hemodialysis patients with comparable lipid control: the Calcium Acetate Renagel Evaluation-2 (CARE-2) study. *Am J Kidney Dis*. 2008;51:952–965.

Slatopolsky E, Robson AM, Elkan I, et al. Control of phosphate excretion in uremic man. *J Clin Invest*. 1968;47:1865–1874.

Stevens LA, Djurdjev O, Cardew S, et al. Calcium, phosphate, and parathyroid hormone levels in combination and as a function of dialysis duration predict mortality: evidence for the complexity of the association between mineral metabolism and outcomes. *J Am Soc Nephrol*. 2004;15:770–779.

Sullivan C, Sayre SS, Leon JB, et al. Effect of food additives on hyperphosphatemia among patients with end-stage renal disease: a randomized controlled trial. *JAMA*. 2009;301:629–635.

Uribarri J, Calvo MS. Hidden sources of phosphorus in the typical American diet: does it matter in nephrology? *Semin Dial*. 2003;16:186–188.

Wada K, Wada Y. Evaluation of aortic calcification with lanthanum carbonate vs. calcium-based phosphate binders in maintenance hemodialysis patients with type 2 diabetes mellitus: an open-label randomized controlled trial. *Ther Apher Dial*. 2014;18:353–360.

Wanner C, Krane V, März W, et al. Atorvastatin in patients with type 2 diabetes mellitus undergoing hemodialysis. *N Engl J Med*. 2005;353:238–248.

Yokoyama K, Hirakata H, Akiba T, et al. Ferric citrate hydrate for the treatment of hyperphosphatemia in nondialysis-dependent CKD. *Clin J Am Soc Nephrol*. 2014;9:543–552.

Young EW, Akiba T, Albert JM, et al. Magnitude and impact of abnormal mineral metabolism in hemodialysis patients in the Dialysis Outcomes and Practice Patterns Study (DOPPS). *Am J Kidney Dis*. 2004;44:34–38.

17

Which Renal Cysts Require Follow-up Evaluation?

With the ubiquitous imaging being performed today, it is very common to discover incidental renal cysts. Clinicians usually turn to nephrologists to ask what to do about them.

CLINICAL AND RADIOLOGIC CHARACTERISTICS

Most renal cysts in adults are simple renal cysts. A cyst is a sac of clear, serous fluid (ultrafiltrate of plasma) that is lined by a single layer of epithelial cells. Renal cysts are derived from progressive dilatation and detachment of diverticula in the distal convoluted tubule and collecting duct. Incidental cysts may be solitary or multiple, and their frequency increases with age. (Up to 50% of patients aged 40–50 years will have cysts.) Patients are usually asymptomatic but rarely may have abdominal or flank discomfort or develop hematuria or symptoms and signs of infection. Hypertension due to cyst compression of normal renal tissue is rare. Diagnosis is generally made as an incidental finding on renal or abdominal ultrasound, computed tomography (CT), or magnetic resonance imaging (MRI).

On renal ultrasound, simple cysts are typically round and sharply demarcated with smooth walls and without echoes within the cyst (Fig. 17.1). Sometimes there may be thin internal septations (Fig 17.2). A strong posterior wall echo indicating good transmission through the cyst and enhanced transmission beyond the cyst are characteristic. Such cysts are benign and do not require follow-up imaging. The primary clinical concern is accurately distinguishing simple renal cysts from complex renal cysts, the latter of which are associated with an increased risk of malignancy and do require follow-up and/or further testing. Some cysts

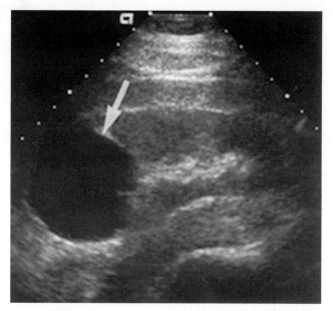

FIGURE 17.1 Simple cyst on renal ultrasound.

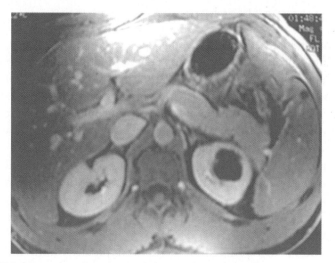

FIGURE 17.2 Septated renal cyst on renal ultrasound.

cannot be characterized noninvasively with certainty, and may require biopsy or surgical excision for diagnosis.

Occasionally, autosomal dominant polycystic kidney disease (PKD) will be discovered on renal imaging; in this disorder, the kidneys will be large (sometimes very large) and filled with innumerable renal cysts. There will generally be a family history of the disorder as well as coexisting liver cysts. Acquired cystic disease, characterized by multiple renal cysts in patients with end-stage renal disease (ESRD), usually after several years of dialysis, can also be easily detected; in this case, the noncystic renal tissue is atrophic. Smaller cysts, usually less than 1 cm in diameter, occur in medullary sponge kidney, autosomal recessive PKD, and autosomal dominant interstitial kidney disease (previously called medullary cystic kidney disease).

When ultrasonography is inconclusive, radiologists generally recommend a renal CT with contrast (unless there is renal failure). CT criteria to distinguish benign from complex cysts have been developed. Using the Bosniak classification, cysts can be classified on the basis of morphologic and contrast enhancement characteristics (Israel and Bosniak, 2005):

> Category I: Benign simple cyst with a thin wall without septa, calcifications, or solid components; water density; no contrast enhancement; no follow-up needed (Fig. 17.3A).

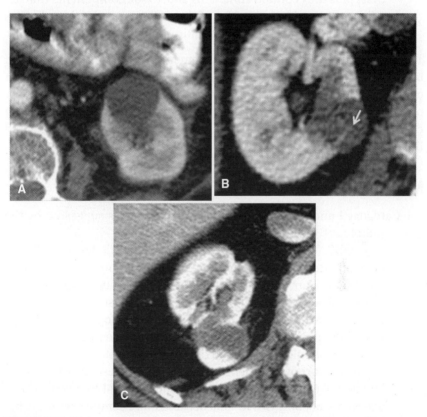

FIGURE 17.3 CT showing a simple category I kidney cyst **(A)**, a simple Category IIF cyst containing thin internal septae (*arrow*) **(B)**, and cystic adenocarcinoma (Category IV cyst) **(C)**.

Category II: Benign cystic lesions in which there may be a few thin septa; the wall or septa may contain fine calcification or a short segment of slightly thickened calcification; less than 3 cm in diameter, well-marginated, no measurable contrast enhancement; no follow-up needed (Fig. 17.3B).

Category IIF: Multiple thin septa or minimal smooth thickening of the septa or wall, which may contain calcification that may also be thick and nodular; no measurable contrast enhancement; may be more than 3 cm in diameter; require follow-up to ascertain that they are nonmalignant.

Category III: Indeterminate cystic masses with thickened irregular or smooth walls or septa; measurable contrast enhancement is present; risk of malignancy is about 50% (cystic renal cell carcinoma and multiloculated cystic renal cell carcinoma); require further imaging and consideration of surgery .

Category IV: These lesions have all the characteristics of category III cysts plus they contain enhancing soft-tissue components that are adjacent to and independent of the wall or septum; these lesions are very likely malignant and require surgery (Fig. 17.3C).

The presence of true contrast enhancement of the lesion (a minimum increased attenuation of 10–15 Hounsfield units) is the most important characteristic separating categories III and IV, which, as noted previously, are associated with malignancy in 50% to 100% of cases, from the categories I, II, and IIF, which are typically benign processes (Israel and Bosniak, 2005).

MANAGEMENT OF RENAL CYSTS

Category I and II: No follow-up is needed (unless suggested by the radiologist!).

Category IIF: The optimal approach to renal cystic lesions with indeterminate findings is uncertain. Examination of prior studies for comparison, if such studies are available, can be very helpful. In their absence, an additional imaging study (such as a contrast-enhanced MRI) is often needed. If the radiologist is unable to clearly distinguish a category IIF lesion from a category III lesion, the lesion should be considered a category III lesion.

In a report of 42 patients with category IIF lesions who had follow-up CT examinations for more than or equal to 2 years (average 5.8 years), only two lesions became more complex with thicker septa; both were found to be cystic neoplasms at surgery (Israel and

Bosniak, 2003). However, in other studies, up to 25% of Bosniak IIF lesions were ultimately found to be malignant (Smith et al., 2012), pointing to the importance of careful follow-up in such patients.

Category III: The approach to category III lesions varies among clinicians. Options include continued surveillance with periodic imaging, fine-needle biopsy, or surgery with partial nephrectomy, if feasible. The best approach depends on the appearance of the lesion and the comorbidities and wishes of the patient. Such lesions are often characterized by MRI and with close surveillance by MRI (typically at 3, 6, and 12 months) (Marotti et al., 1987; Israel et al., 2004). Further imaging is generally not necessary if the cysts are stable at 12 months. MRI is most useful for characterizing the internal contents of cysts, such as hemorrhage or mucin, and is more sensitive than both ultrasound and CT in showing enhancement of internal septations, which suggests the presence of malignancy. In one study, 37 patients with 55 complex cystic renal lesions underwent T1-weighted, T2-weighted, and gadolinium-enhanced MRI (Balci et al., 1999). The combination of mural irregularity and intense mural enhancement had the highest correlation with malignancy.

Percutaneous needle biopsy can provide a diagnosis in up to 80% of cases. An important caveat is that failure to make a definite diagnosis (either benign or malignant) still leaves open the possibility of an undiagnosed malignancy. In one study of 583 patients in whom image-guided biopsy was performed for indeterminate renal lesions, a diagnosis was made in only 76% (Richter et al., 2000).

Category IV: Category IV lesions require surgery, since approximately 85% to 100% are malignant (Israel and Bosniak, 2005).

EPIDEMIOLOGY

The prevalence of simple renal cysts varies with the population studied and the imaging modality utilized. These cysts occur most often in patients more than 50 years of age and are more common in men than women. In the largest reported study, in which 14,314 Japanese individuals underwent a screening program, at least one renal cyst was found on ultrasonography in 12% (Terada et al., 2008). The incidence of cysts was twofold higher in men compared with women, and the prevalence increased from 5% to 36% from the fourth to the eighth decade of life. Interestingly, cyst growth was faster in younger patients ($<$50 years of age).

IS THERE ANY CHANCE THAT A SIMPLE CYST IS HARBORING A MALIGNANCY?

An older retrospective study assessed 260 lesions detected by intravenous pyelography in 242 patients; subsequent renal ultrasound was performed, with the ultrasonographic diagnosis confirmed by cyst puncture, surgery, or autopsy (Clayman et al., 1984). Of the 260 lesions, 168 were benign cysts, and all were diagnosed correctly by ultrasonography. The remaining 92 lesions were renal carcinomas, 90 of which were diagnosed correctly by ultrasonography. The two missed cancers did not meet all three ultrasonographic criteria for a benign cyst (Clayman et al., 1984). Therefore, clear-cut simple cysts are rarely, if ever, malignant and do not require follow-up imaging.

PATIENT 1

A 75-year-old man undergoes renal ultrasonography because of the finding of chronic kidney disease (CKD). A large simple cyst is found in the right kidney.

Q: What is your next step?

1. Follow-up ultrasound in 6 months
2. Follow-up ultrasound in 12 months
3. CT scan with contrast for further evaluation
4. No follow-up needed

A: The correct answer is (4). Simple cysts are common in elderly male patients and, regardless of the size, are exceedingly unlikely to be malignant or develop into a malignancy.

PATIENT 2

A 45-year-old woman is seen by a nephrologist because of hypertension and CKD. She has a strong family history of PKD (father, paternal uncle, and sister all were diagnosed with the disease, with her father and uncle requiring dialysis). Renal ultrasound reveals bilaterally large (15 cm) kidneys filled with innumerable cysts.

Q: Which of the following are true statements?

1. A CT scan with contrast should be periodically performed to assess for malignant transformation of cysts
2. Hypertension is likely due to compression of normal renal tissue by the cysts, leading to stimulation of the renin–angiotensin system
3. The kidneys are likely to continue to grow in size
4. Lack of symptoms related to the cystic kidneys is decidedly unusual

A: The correct answers are (2) and (3). Almost all patients with PKD are hypertensive, and stimulation of the renin–angiotensin system is believed to be the primary mechanism. The kidneys will, in most cases, continue to increase in size as the patient ages. In some patients, they may become large enough to lead to abdominal fullness, pain, and even early satiety. Other patients may have hematuria or symptoms of cyst infection. However, many patients remain asymptomatic. PKD is not a premalignant condition, and screening for malignancy is unnecessary in the absence of suggestive symptoms and signs. The possible presence of an underlying malignancy should be suspected if there is fever, anorexia, fatigue, and weight loss that cannot be explained by severity of the renal disease or renal infection, or if there is rapid growth of a complex cyst.

References

Balci NC, Semelka RC, Patt RH, et al. Complex renal cysts: findings on MR imaging. *Am J Roentgenol.* 1999;172:1495.

Clayman RV, Surya V, Miller RP, et al. Pursuit of the renal mass. Is ultrasound enough? *Am J Med.* 1984;77:218.

Israel GM, Bosniak MA. Follow-up CT of moderately complex cystic lesions of the kidney (Bosniak category IIF). *Am J Roentgenol.* 2003;181:627.

Israel GM, Bosniak MA. An update of the Bosniak renal cyst classification system. *Urology.* 2005;66:484.

Israel GM, Hindman N, Bosniak MA. Evaluation of cystic renal masses: comparison of CT and MR imaging by using the Bosniak classification system. *Radiology.* 2004;231:365.

Marotti M, Hricak H, Fritzsche P, et al. Complex and simple renal cysts: comparative evaluation with MR imaging. *Radiology.* 1987;162:679.

Richter F, Kasabian NG, Irwin RJ Jr, et al. Accuracy of diagnosis by guided biopsy of renal mass lesions classified indeterminate by imaging studies. *Urology.* 2000;55:348.

Smith AD, Remer EM, Cox KL, et al. Bosniak category IIF and III cystic renal lesions: outcomes and associations. *Radiology.* 2012;262:152.

Terada N, Ichioka K, Matsuta Y, et al. The natural history of simple renal cysts. *J Urol.* 2002;167:21.

18

Are Renin–Angiotensin–Aldosterone System Blockers Friends or Foes of the Kidneys?

The renin–angiotensin–aldosterone system (RAAS) plays an important role in the regulation of systemic volume homeostasis and blood pressure (BP). The classic systemic RAAS is depicted in Figure 18.1. In addition, there is an intrarenal RAAS that controls glomerular capillary pressure and glomerular filtration (Fig. 18.2). There is also evolving evidence for the existence of an intracellular RAAS, as angiotensin II (Ang II) and aldosterone are capable of stimulating various cellular processes, including growth factors and reactive oxygen species, which can lead to fibrosis (Leehey et al., 2006; Bertocchio et al., 2011).

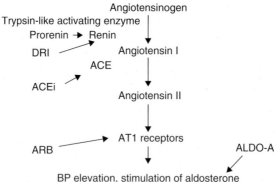

FIGURE 18.1 The systemic RAAS depicting the site of action of direct renin inhibitors (DRIs), ACE inhibitors (ACEis), ARBs, and aldosterone antagonists (ALDO-As).

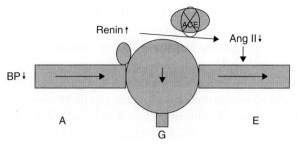

FIGURE 18.2 The intrarenal RAAS, depicting the effect on the renal circulation of lowering BP with an ACE inhibitor. Renin secretion will be increased due to the decrease in pressure and flow in the afferent arteriole (*A*), but since conversion of angiotensin I to angiotensin II (Ang II) is inhibited, there will be less Ang II–mediated constriction of the efferent arteriole (*E*) and a fall in glomerular (*G*) capillary pressure will occur. (From Moinuddin IK, Leehey DJ. *Handbook of Nephrology.* Philadelphia, PA: Lippincott Williams & Wilkins; 2013.)

Experimental work in the 1980s provided evidence that blockade of the RAAS with angiotensin-converting enzyme (ACE) inhibitors could prevent glomerulosclerosis and progressive renal failure in animal models of kidney disease, and in particular, diabetic kidney disease (Zatz et al., 1986). These observations were followed by clinical trials suggesting a renoprotective effect of ACE inhibitors, which is, at least in part, independent of their effects on BP (Lewis et al., 1993). The mechanism of renal benefit may be explained by the observation that Ang II can preferentially constrict the efferent versus the afferent arterioles in the kidney; prevention of Ang II formation or action therefore decreases glomerular capillary pressure (Fig. 18.2). A hemodynamically mediated renoprotective effect of RAAS blockers is suggested from observations that these agents appear to preferentially decrease proteinuria when compared to other antihypertensive agents. A decrease in proteinuria has been used as surrogate of renal protection in many studies, as interventions that decrease proteinuria generally result in more favorable renal outcomes. However, there are exceptions to this, which can particularly be seen in studies where combined RAAS blockade was utilized for the treatment of diabetic kidney disease. For instance, in the Veterans Affairs Nephropathy in Diabetes Trial (VA NEPHRON-D) trial, dual RAAS blockade with the ACE inhibitor lisinopril and the angiotensin receptor blocker (ARB) losartan decreased proteinuria more than monotherapy with losartan alone; however, this did not lead to a statistically significant reduction in hard renal endpoints and was associated with a greater risk of adverse events including AKI and hyperkalemia (Fried et al., 2013).

Clinical trials comparing RAAS blockers to other antihypertensive agents have generally reported lower BPs in patients treated with RAAS blockers. An exception was the Irbesartan Diabetic Nephropathy Trial (IDN) study, in which the ARB irbesartan was compared to amlodipine, a dihydropyridine calcium channel blocker (Lewis et al., 2001). In this study, despite similar BP control in the two arms, patients receiving the ARB had better renal outcomes. However, it should be pointed out that dihydropyridine calcium channel blockers can increase glomerular capillary pressure because of dilation of the afferent arteriole. Thus, a possible interpretation of the IDNT study is that calcium blockers have adverse renal effects rather than RAAS inhibitors having beneficial renal effects. In a recent meta-analysis, it was reported that RAAS blockers do not prolong survival in patients with diabetic kidney disease; however, they did appear to decrease end-stage kidney disease (Palmer et al., 2015).

Evidence supports using ACE inhibitors or ARBs as primary agents to reduce risk of chronic kidney disease (CKD) progression in patients with CKD, and in particular patients with proteinuric diabetic kidney disease (Cao et al., 2012; Ruggenenti et al., 2012). However, use of RAAS agents in such patients is not without risks (St Peter et al., 2013). Because of their intrarenal hemodynamic effects, that is, lowering of glomerular capillary pressure, use of RAAS blockers, although protective in the long term, will increase the risk of an acute decline in renal function. Excessive reduction in GFR can occur with their use, in particular when there is actual or effective volume depletion or if used with other drugs that affect interglomerular hemodynamics (e.g., nonsteroidal anti-inflammatory drugs, contrast media) or in the presence of bilateral renal artery stenosis. Moreover, because of inhibition of aldosterone release or blockade of its receptors, there is a risk of hyperkalemia. An acute decrease in renal function will also predispose to development of hyperkalemia. The risk of hyperkalemia is a particular concern in diabetic patients, as many such patients have a tendency to be hyperkalemic even in the absence of RAAS inhibition due to both a defect in insulin-mediated potassium transport into cells and underlying hypoaldosteronism.

In view of these known adverse effects of RAAS blockers, and in view of physicians desire to do no harm, clinicians frequently wonder if the benefits of RAAS blockers outweigh the risk in patients with CKD. There have been few studies designed to address this issue. Stopping RAAS inhibitors can increase estimated glomerular filtration rate (eGFR) in a substantial number of advanced CKD patients. In one study of 43 stage 4 CKD (eGFR 15–30 mL/min/1.73 m^2) patients, those who had eGFR improvement of more than or equal to 5 mL/min/1.73 m^2 after drug cessation were the most likely to survive long term without dialysis (Gonçalves et al., 2011). On the other hand, others believe that many patients with advanced CKD who could benefit from RAAS blockers are not receiving them (Shirazian et al., 2015).

Several precautions should be taken to try to prevent the development of acute renal failure and hyperkalemia in patients receiving RAAS inhibitors. BP goals should be individualized, with avoidance of low BP (<120/60 mm Hg), especially in the elderly. Dual RAAS inhibitor therapy should rarely, if ever, be employed. RAAS blockers should be avoided in patients with hyperkalemia or with diagnosed or suspected bilateral renal artery stenosis.

Specific recommendations concerning monitoring of serum creatinine and potassium levels in patients receiving RAAS blockers are given in Table 18.1. These recommendations are adapted from the protocol of the VA NEPHRON-D study. It should be remembered however that despite protocols to decrease the likelihood of acute renal failure or hyperkalemia, the VA NEPHRON-D study was stopped early because of increased risk of these complications. Therefore, in clinical practice, it is probably prudent to be even more conservative with the use of RAAS inhibitors than outlined in the table.

In summary, it is clear that RAAS therapy can be a double-edged sword in CKD management, particularly in diabetic patients. Evidence

TABLE 18.1 Management of the Patient Taking RAAS Inhibitors

Prevention of AKI

1. Check serum creatinine concentration within 2 wk of initiating a RAAS inhibitor or increasing the dose of a RAAS inhibitor. If the serum creatinine increases >30% from baseline, decrease the dose (or stop the drug if at lowest dose).
2. Adjust diuretic dose as necessary and assure that the patient is not taking nonsteroidal anti-inflammatory drugs.

Prevention of Hyperkalemia

1. Do not start RAAS inhibitors unless serum potassium concentration is <5 mmol/L. This can generally be achieved with use of a low potassium diet and diuretics.
2. If the serum potassium level is >5 mmol/L, assure a low potassium diet and increase diuretics if indicated.
3. If the serum potassium level increases to >5.5 mmol/L, in addition to the measures shown in (2), administration of long-term alkali supplements, liberalizing salt intake (if not contraindicated), or use of a potassium binding agent may be indicated.
4. If the serum potassium level increases to >6 mmol/L, stop the RAAS inhibitor. The RAAS inhibitor may be reinstituted at 50% of the prior dose once serum potassium is <5.5 mmol/L.
5. If serum potassium increases to >6.5 mmol/L, permanently discontinue the RAAS inhibitor.

shows that RAAS inhibitors can slow progression of both diabetic and nondiabetic CKD; however, overly aggressive use in patients at risk for adverse effects and/or inadequate monitoring can result in situations where the risk outweighs the benefit.

PATIENT 1

A 50-year-old Caucasian man with a long history of diabetes and hypertension is seen in the clinic. On examination, he has a BP 160/100 mm Hg and 2+ lower extremity edema. His urinalysis shows 3+ protein and no cells. His serum creatinine is 1.6 mg/dL, his serum potassium is 4.4 mmol/L, and his eGFR is 49 mL/min/1.73 m^2. He is started on a diuretic and losartan. Two weeks later, his serum creatinine is 2 mg/dL and his serum potassium is 5.2 mmol/L. His BP is now 135/80 mm Hg and his edema is improved.

Q: What is the best course of action?

1. Stop the losartan
2. Stop the diuretic
3. Counsel the patient on a low potassium diet
4. Continue current management

A: The increase in serum creatinine is likely due to the institution of the diuretic and ARB, which have led to a decrease in glomerular capillary pressure and glomerular filtration. The increase in serum creatinine is only 25%, so there is no need to stop losartan or decrease the dose. Stopping the diuretic will result in return of edema and possibly result in hyperkalemia. However, the serum potassium is now greater than 5 mmol/L, so a low potassium diet is necessary.

PATIENT 2

A 60-year-old Caucasian man with a long history of hypertension and tobacco use is seen in the clinic because of uncontrolled BP. His BP is 170/100 mm Hg and he is started on the ACE inhibitor lisinopril. Two weeks later, he returns for a nurse visit to have his BP checked and laboratory tests repeated. His serum creatinine has increased from 1.2 to 2 mg/dL during the two-week interval. His BP is now 150/90 mm Hg.

Q: What is the best course of action?

1. Stop the lisinopril
2. Increase the lisinopril
3. Continue current management
4. Performed a duplex ultrasound of the renal arteries

A: The correct answers are (1) and (4). The marked increase in serum creatinine after starting a RAAS inhibitor without much about decrease in BP suggests the possibility of bilateral renal artery stenosis. In most institutions, the first test to perform would be a duplex study of the renal arteries. However, other alternatives in this case would be CT angiography, MRA of the renal arteries with or without contrast depending on the serum creatinine, or if the index of suspicion is very high, renal angiography.

References

Bertocchio JP, Warnock DG, Jaisser F. Mineralocorticoid receptor activation and blockade: an emerging paradigm in chronic kidney disease. *Kidney Int.* 2011;79(10):1051–1060.

Cao Z, Cooper ME. Efficacy of renin-angiotensin system (RAS) blockers on cardiovascular and renal outcomes in patients with type 2 diabetes. *Acta Diabetol.* 2012;49(4):243–254.

Fried LF, Emanuele N, Zhang JH, et al.; for the VA NEPHRON-D Investigators. Combined angiotensin inhibition for treatment of diabetic nephropathy. *N Engl J Med.* 2013;369(20):1892–1903.

Gonçalves AR, Khwaja A, Ahmed AK, et al. Stopping renin-angiotensin system inhibitors in chronic kidney disease: predictors of response. *Nephron Clin Pract.* 2011;119(4):c348–c354.

Leehey DJ, Singh AK, Singh R. Angiotensin II and its receptors in diabetic nephropathy. In: Mogensen CE, Cortes P, eds. *The Diabetic Kidney*. Totowa, NJ: Humana Press; 2006.

Lewis EJ, Hunsicker LG, Bain RP, et al.; The Collaborative Study Group. The effect of angiotensin-converting-enzyme inhibition on diabetic nephropathy. *N Engl J Med.* 1993;329(20):1456–1462.

Lewis EJ, Hunsicker LG, Clarke WR, et al.; The Collaborative Study Group. Renoprotective effect of the angiotensin-receptor antagonist irbesartan in patients with nephropathy due to type 2 diabetes. *N Engl J Med.* 2001;345(12):851–860.

Palmer SC, Mavridis D, Navarese E, et al. Comparative efficacy and safety of blood pressure-lowering agents in adults with diabetes and kidney disease: a network meta-analysis. *Lancet.* 2015;385(9982):2047–2056.

Ruggenenti P, Cravedi P, Remuzzi G. Mechanisms and treatment of CKD. *J Am Soc Nephrol.* 2012;23(12):1917–1928.

Shirazian S, Grant CD, Mujeeb S, et al. Underprescription of renin-angiotensin system blockers in moderate to severe chronic kidney disease. *Am J Med Sci.* 2015;349(6):510–515.

St Peter WL, Odum LE, Whaley-Connell AT. To RAS or not to RAS? The evidence for and cautions with renin-angiotensin system inhibition in patients with diabetic kidney disease. *Pharmacotherapy.* 2013;33(5):496–514.

Zatz R, Dunn BR, Meyer TW, et al. Prevention of diabetic glomerulopathy by pharmacological amelioration of glomerular capillary hypertension. *J Clin Invest.* 1986;77(6):1925–1930.

Does a Patient with a Mild Decrease in Estimated Glomerular Filtration Rate Really Have a Disease?

All clinical laboratories now report a measure of estimated glomerular filtration rate (eGFR) when they report serum creatinine. There are several eGFR formulae now available. The original ones were developed from data obtained in the Modification of Diet in Renal Disease (MDRD) Study. Since this study did not include many non-Caucasian or diabetic patients, and was based on subjects with fairly advanced renal failure, the CKD-EPI (Chronic Kidney Disease Epidemiology Collaboration) equation was subsequently developed on the basis of data from several clinical trials including a much broader range of patients, and is more applicable to patients with normal or near-normal renal function. These estimating equations use serum creatinine along with some combination of age, sex, race, and body size as surrogates for the non-GFR determinants of serum creatinine. Subsequently, other formulae using measures of cystatin C, instead of or in addition to creatinine, have been used by some laboratories. Cystatin C may have advantages over creatinine for GFR estimation because its non-GFR determinants are less affected by race and muscle mass. Use of cystatin C and creatinine together may allow more accurate GFR estimates, but such equations are not in common use. Regardless of which formula is used, there are many patients who are reported to have an eGFR of less than 60 mL/min/1.73 m^2, and thus are labelled as having stage 3 CKD (see Table 4.1). Do they really have a disease?

The staging system for CKD was developed to aid clinicians in the management of patients with kidney disease by identifying those with the most severe disease who are at greatest risk for progression and complications. Using current definitions, the prevalence of CKD in the United States during the interval from 1999 to 2006 was 11.5%, and the prevalence of CKD in people 70 years and older in the United States was approximately 45% (Levey, 2009). This is a very large percentage of elderly persons now being labelled with a disease.

The association between older age and lower eGFR in cross-sectional studies has traditionally been thought to be due to a natural aging process, with GFR typically declining at a rate of about 1 mL/min/year after the age of 40 years (Lindeman and Goldman, 1986). However, the observation that some individuals followed longitudinally do not lose kidney function as they age suggests that involutional changes due to aging alone do not completely explain the lower eGFR seen in elderly patients in cross-sectional studies. Moreover, lower eGFR values are associated with kidney as well as cardiovascular disease in older as well as younger individuals, suggesting that decreased eGFR in the elderly is evidence of disease. Similarly, the increased risk for individuals with albuminuria in older as well as younger adults suggests that albuminuria is also indicative of a disease in patients regardless of age (Hallan et al., 2012).

Whether or not a mild decrease in eGFR is really a disease, there is little doubt that ubiquitous reporting of eGFR has led to an increase in nephrology consultations for mild decreases in eGFR, especially in older individuals. In the majority of such instances, specialist referral is unnecessary. Most guidelines suggest that patients with severely decreased GFR (eGFR <30 mL/min/1.73 m^2, i.e., CKD stage 4) should be referred for comanagement with a nephrologist, since such patients have progressive kidney disease and are at high risk for progression to end-stage renal disease (ESRD). In the event that they eventually require dialysis, it has been demonstrated that late referral to a nephrologist is associated with higher mortality after the initiation of dialysis (Kinchen et al., 2002). There is less consensus about referral for patients with higher eGFR. Kidney Disease: Improving Global Outcomes (K-DIGO) guidelines recommend that in those with eGFR more than 30 mL/min/1.73 m^2, the following features should generally prompt nephrology referral (KDIGO, 2013):

- Urine albumin-to-creatinine ratio (ACR) more than or equal to 300 mg/g (34 mg/mmol)
- Hematuria not secondary to urological conditions
- Inability to identify a presumed cause of CKD
- Rapid eGFR decline without an obvious explanation

- Presence of complications of CKD, such as anemia requiring erythro-poietin therapy and abnormalities of bone and mineral metabolism requiring phosphorus binders or vitamin D preparations
- Persistent hyperkalemia
- Resistant hypertension
- Recurrent or extensive nephrolithiasis
- Confirmed or presumed hereditary kidney disease
- Patients under the age of 18 years

PATIENT 1

A 75-year-old man with mild essential hypertension and osteoarthritis is seen by his internist for a routine examination. Medications include chlorthalidone, tramadol, and vitamins. He does not take nonsteroidal anti-inflammatory drugs. Physical examination reveals a blood pressure of 138/72 mm Hg and mild arthritic changes in the hands. Laboratory review reveals an eGFR of 56 mL/min/1.73 m^2. Urinalysis reveals no proteinuria. Review of past laboratory results indicates that the eGFR has been in this range for the past several years.

Q: Does this patient require referral to a nephrologist?

A: This elderly gentleman has well-controlled blood pressure and a minimal decrease in eGFR that has been stable for several years. He is extremely unlikely to ever develop ESRD in view of his age, absence of proteinuria, and lack of progression. He does not require nephrology referral.

PATIENT 2

A 55-year-old man with no significant past medical history is seen by an internist because of low-grade fever, 20 pound weight loss, arthralgias, and a skin rash. He is taking no medications and denies the use of over-the-counter medications. He is normotensive and has a temperature of 38°C. He has a palpable purpuric rash on the lower extremities. The remaining of the examination is normal. His eGFR is 56 mL/min/1.73 m^2. Urinalysis reveals 2+ proteinuria and 10 to 20 red blood cells per high-power field. There are no previous laboratory values available.

Q: Does this patient require referral to a nephrologist?

A: The presence of systemic symptoms and hematuria and proteinuria on urinalysis coupled with the mild decrease in eGFR suggest the presence of a systemic disease involving the kidneys such as vasculitis or glomerulonephritis. This patient requires prompt nephrology referral.

References

Hallan SI, Matsushita K, Sang Y, et al.; Chronic Kidney Disease Prognosis Consortium. Age and association of kidney measures with mortality and end-stage renal disease. *JAMA.* 2012;308(22):2349–2360.

KDIGO. Chapter 1: definition and classification of CKD. *Kidney Int Suppl.* 2013;3:19. http://www .kdigo.org/clinical_practice_guidelines/pdf/CKD/KDIGO_2012_CKD_GL.pdf.

Kinchen KS, Sadler J, Fink N, et al. The timing of specialist evaluation in chronic kidney disease and mortality. *Ann Intern Med.* 2002;137:479.

Levey AS, Stevens LA, Schmid CH, et al. A new equation to estimate glomerular filtration rate. *Ann Intern Med.* 2009;150(9):604–612.

Lindeman RD, Goldman R. Anatomic and physiologic age changes in the kidney. *Exp Gerontol.* 1986;21(4/5):379–406.

Why Are Kidney Stones a Nephrologic As Well As a Urologic Disease?

Kidney stones (nephrolithiasis) will occur in 12% of men and 5% of women during their lifetime. Thus, this is a very common disease. The major types of stones are calcium (70%–80%, oxalate more common than phosphate), uric acid (5%–10%), cystine (<1%), and magnesium ammonium phosphate (struvite) (10%). Combined calcium/urate stones are also often seen. A patient with a calcium-containing stone episode has an overall 50% chance of recurrence within 10 years, which is higher for men than for women. Some patients will have many recurrent stones, leading to substantial morbidity, medical costs, and even mortality. Yet too many nonnephrologists continue to view stone disease as a urologic, that is, surgical, disease rather than a nephrologic, that is, medical, disease. This is very unfortunate, as medical therapy can substantially lower the risk of recurrent stones.

Most kidney stones contain calcium. Idiopathic hypercalciuria is the most common etiology of calcium stones. This is a multigenic autosomal dominant disease. The exact pathogenesis is uncertain, and may have different etiologies in different patients, which include renal phosphorus and/or calcium leak, intestinal hyperabsorption, and increased bone resorption. Risk factors for calcium stones include higher urinary calcium excretion (Marshall et al., 1972), lower urinary volume, higher urinary oxalate excretion (calcium oxalate stones), higher urinary uric acid excretion (uric acid serves as a nidus for calcium stone formation), lower urinary citrate excretion (citrate is a stone inhibitor), higher urinary pH (calcium phosphate stones form in alkaline urine), and anatomic

	Risk Factors for Calcium Stone Formation

- Hypercalciuria—61%, including some patients with primary hyperparathyroidism
- Hyperuricosuria—36%
- Hypocitraturia—28% idiopathic and 3.3% due to type 1 (distal) renal tubular acidosis (RTA) or chronic diarrhea
- Low urine volume (<1 L/day)—15%
- Hyperoxaluria—8%, including enteric and primary forms and markedly increased oxalate intake

Reprinted from Levy FL, Adams-Huet B, Pak CY. Ambulatory evaluation of nephrolithiasis: an update of a 1980 protocol. *Am J Med.* 1995;98(1):50–59, with permission from Elsevier.

abnormalities (medullary sponge kidney, horseshoe kidney). In one study, over 60% of patients with calcium stones had hypercalciuria, over one-third had hyperuricosuria and over one-fourth had hypocitraturia (Levy et al., 1995) (Table 20.1).

EVALUATION OF PATIENTS WITH RECURRENT KIDNEY STONES

Patients with recurrent calcium stones require metabolic evaluation to detect biochemical abnormalities, which, if corrected, will lessen the chance of recurrence. Of course, hypercalcemia should be excluded, as such patients are generally also hypercalciuric and treatment of the etiology of hypercalcemia should correct the stone problem. Occasionally, patients may have an underlying distal renal tubular acidosis (RTA), resulting in bone resorption and hypercalciuria. A clue to the presence of RTA is the development of calcium phosphate rather than calcium oxalate stones, which are preferentially formed when the urine pH is elevated. Enteric hyperoxaluria can be seen in malabsorption syndromes such as inflammatory bowel disease and after bariatric surgery. In this disorder, fat malabsorption results in increased binding of calcium to fat and decreased binding of calcium to oxalate in the gut, resulting in more free oxalate available for absorption by the colon; in addition, bile salt–induced increase in colonic oxalate absorption contributes to hyperoxaluria (Smith et al., 1972; Chadwick et al., 1973; Nasr et al., 2008).

Determination of the type of stone and evaluation for biochemical abnormalities or underlying conditions that predispose to stone formation are essential for guiding therapy to prevent recurrent disease. Spontaneously passed or surgically removed stones should undergo stone

TABLE 20.2   Dietary Risk Factors for Calcium Stones

- Lower dietary calcium (increases oxalate absorption and urinary oxalate excretion)
- Higher dietary oxalate (increases urinary oxalate excretion)
- Lower dietary potassium (may increase urinary calcium excretion)
- Higher animal protein intake (increases calcium and uric acid excretion, lowers urine pH thus decreasing citrate excretion)
- Higher sodium intake (increases calcium excretion)
- Higher sucrose intake (may increase calcium excretion)
- High vitamin C intake (increases oxalate excretion)
- High vitamin D intake (increases calcium excretion)

TABLE 20.3   Characteristics of Patients at High Risk for Recurrent Stones

Middle-aged, white males with a family history of stones (likely hypercalciuria)
Pathologic skeletal fractures or osteoporosis (likely hypercalciuria)
Recurrent urinary tract infections (possible struvite stones)
Gout (likely hyperuricosuria)
Chronic diarrheal states and/or malabsorption (possible enteric hyperoxaluria)
Stone analysis revealing cystine, uric acid, calcium phosphate, or struvite stones

analysis. Patients presenting with their first stone require a careful dietary history (Table 20.2) and a limited laboratory evaluation to exclude hypercalcemia (such as with primary hyperparathyroidism) or hyperchloremic acidosis (such as with distal RTA). A complete metabolic evaluation is indicated in patients with recurrent stones or multiple stones at first presentation (for instance, a stone passage episode accompanied by one or more stones seen in the kidneys on imaging studies). Patients with a strong family history of stones should also undergo a complete metabolic evaluation, as such patients are likely to have idiopathic hypercalciuria. Some have also a recommended a complete metabolic evaluation in patient at high risk for recurrent stone formation (Preminger, 1989) (Table 20.3).

COMPLETE METABOLIC EVALUATION

The complete metabolic evaluation for nephrolithiasis consists of both blood and urine testing, and should include at least two 24-hour urine collections (Table 20.4). This test is now standardized in most clinical laboratories, with most using a reference laboratory that provides a

TABLE 20.4	Complete Metabolic Evaluation for Nephrolithiasis

Blood

Serum calcium (if elevated, suggests primary hyperparathyroidism or other cause of hypercalcemia)

Serum electrolytes (low total CO_2 raises the possibility of distal RTA)

Urine

Urinalysis—urine pH >7 with phosphate crystals in the urine sediment suggests calcium phosphate or struvite stones (struvite stones have a typical coffin-lid appearance); hexagonal cystine crystals are diagnostic of cystinuria; other crystals (calcium, uric acid, indinavir, etc.) may suggest etiology of stones

24-hour urine collection(s) for urine stone risk diagnostic profile. This test is now standardized in most clinical laboratories, with most using a reference laboratory that provides a graphical display of results (see Fig. 20.1)

graphical display of results (Pak et al., 1985). An example of a graphical display is shown in Figure 20.1.

TREATMENT OF CALCIUM STONES

Treatment of recurrent calcium stones begins with an assessment of dietary habits and correction of dietary risk factors (Table 20.2). Lower fluid intake will increase urinary calcium concentrations, and high fluid intake can help prevent these stones. Decreasing dietary calcium is not recommended since it will actually increase oxalate absorption and urinary oxalate excretion due to less binding of calcium to oxalate in the gut. Avoiding high oxalate foods may be of benefit by decreasing urinary oxalate excretion. Higher dietary potassium may decrease urinary calcium excretion. Limiting animal protein intake will reduce calcium and especially uric acid excretion and also increase citrate excretion. Limiting sodium intake will decrease calcium excretion. There is also some evidence that limiting sucrose intake may decrease calcium excretion. Hyperuricosuria (gout, high animal protein intake) predisposes to calcium stones because uric acid can serve as nidus for calcium stone formation. Mixed calcium/urate stones as well as pure uric acid stones can also occur (Coe et al., 1975). Increased fluid intake will help to prevent calcium stones (Pak et al., 1980). Thus, there is evidence that the common recommendation to drink more fluids is indeed beneficial. (This is one of the few medical situations where drinking a lot of fluids has been proven to have a therapeutic effect.) Decreased protein and sodium intake have

Diagnostic profile

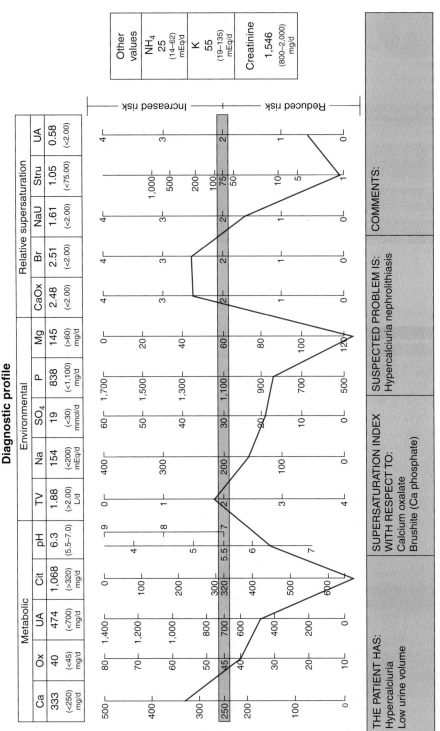

FIGURE 20.1 A sample urine stone risk diagnostic profile. The *gray horizontal bar* in the middle of the figure depicts the upper or lower range of normal for each analyte; abnormal findings appear above the *horizontal bar*. In this patient, hypercalciuria accompanied by relative supersaturation of the urine for calcium oxalate and brushite (calcium phosphate) were present. Ca, calcium; Ox, oxalate; UA, uric acid; Cit, citrate; TV, total (urine) volume; Na, sodium; SO₄, sulfate; P, phosphorus; Mg, magnesium; CaOx, calcium oxalate; Br, brushite; NaU, sodium urate; Stru, struvite; NH, ammonium; K, potassium.

also shown benefit (Muldowney et al., 1982). Thiazide diuretics decrease urinary calcium excretion and should be used in hypercalciuric patients at high risk for recurrence, having coexistent medical conditions (such as hypertension), or recurrent/multiple stones (Laerum and Larsen, 1984). Potassium citrate should be used if urinary citrate is low (Ettinger et al., 1997). Addition of potassium citrate to a thiazide regimen will help prevent diuretic-induced hypokalemia. Allopurinol is indicated if there is coexistent hyperuricosuria unresponsive to dietary restriction (Ettinger et al., 1986).

TREATMENT OF URIC ACID STONES

Risk factors for uric acid stones include low urine pH (often from ingestion of animal proteins) and low urine volume. Some but not all patients will have gout and/or hyperuricosuria (Yü and Gutman, 1967). Since urate (which is quite soluble) and uric acid (which is not, and forms crystals and stones) are in equal concentrations at a urine pH of 5.75 (i.e. the pK for uric acid), measures for prevention and treatment of uric acid stones are to raise the urine pH to more than 6.5 with alkali (Pak et al., 1986) and to increase fluid intake, which will decrease urine uric acid concentration.

TREATMENT OF CYSTINE STONES

Since cystine also precipitates in concentrated acidic urine, urinary alkalinization and increasing urine volume are also beneficial in this rare disease.

TREATMENT OF STRUVITE STONES

Struvite stones are also called infection stones (Rodman, 1999). They are composed of calcium carbonate-apatite and magnesium ammonium phosphate, and form only in the presence of urea-splitting organisms. When urine is infected with such organisms, urea is split into ammonia and carbon dioxide, resulting in alkaline urine that promotes calcium phosphate or magnesium ammonium phosphate crystallization. These stones tend to be of the staghorn variety, are difficult to eradicate even with interventional/surgical procedures, and can cause end-stage kidney disease. They are a known complication of patients with urinary diversion after cystectomy. Patients with struvite stones should have a metabolic evaluation to exclude coexisting hypercalciuria, hypocitraturia, or hyperuricosuria.

PATIENT 1

A 50-year-old white male construction worker with a long history of back pains underwent magnetic resonance imaging, which disclosed renal calculi. He was referred to a urologist, where computed tomography (CT) revealed bilateral stones. He underwent extracorporeal shock wave lithotripsy (ESWL) on two occasions. Stone analysis on the gravel obtained after ESWL showed calcium oxalate. He was subsequently referred by the urologist to a nephrologist. Family history was remarkable for a brother and a cousin with stones. Medications included occasional acetaminophen. Diet was only remarkable for a recent decrease in dairy product intake. There was no history of gout or diarrhea. Physical examination was entirely normal. Plasma electrolytes, urea nitrogen, creatinine, and total calcium (×3) were normal. Urinalysis showed calcium oxalate crystals. A 24-hour urine for stone risk diagnostic profile revealed hypercalciuria (258 mg/24 hours). There was no hyperuricosuria, hypocitraturia, or hyperoxaluria. Urine volume was 1.1 L/day. A repeat urine profile revealed similar findings.

Q: What is the most likely reason for stones in this patient?

1. Idiopathic hypercalciuria
2. Low urine volume
3. No metabolic disorder
4. 1 and 2

A: This patient has a strong family history of stones and a 24-hour urine calcium that is above the normal range. He also has a low urine volume, which means that his urine is likely substantially supersaturated with respect to calcium oxalate. These findings suggest idiopathic hypercalciuria. He was treated with hydrochlorothiazide 25 mg daily to decrease calcium excretion and was also instructed to decrease his sodium and protein intake and to increase his fluid intake. These measures prevented stone recurrence.

PATIENT 2

A 60-year-old white man was admitted for a nasal polypectomy. Eleven years previously, he had donated his left kidney to a brother suffering from end-stage kidney disease. There was no personal or family history of nephrolithiasis or gout. Physical examination revealed nasal polyps and mild hypertension. The plasma urea nitrogen and creatinine were 125 mg/dL (urea 44.6 mmol/L) and 12 mg/dL (1,061 µmol/L), respectively. Urinalysis revealed a urine pH of 5 and numerous uric acid crystals. Plasma uric acid was 8.7 mg/dL (517 µmol/L). Plasma calcium and phosphorus were 9.3 mg/dL (2.3 mmol/L) and 8.2 mg/dL (2.6 mmol/L), respectively. Ultrasound of the solitary right kidney revealed hydronephrosis and multiple stones. Retrograde pyelography showed three radiolucent stones almost obstructing the ureter. A ureteral stent was placed, and the renal pelvis was irrigated with sodium bicarbonate. The stones resolved and the plasma urea nitrogen and creatinine decreased to 14 and 1.4 mg/dL, respectively.

Q: What is the best treatment to prevent recurrence of uric acid stones in this patient?

1. Alkalinization of the urine
2. Increase in fluid intake
3. Allopurinol
4. 1 and 2
5. All of the above

A: Uric acid stones form in concentrated acidic urine, so an increase in fluid intake and urine alkalinization are indicated. The patient was treated with sodium citrate and nightly acetazolamide to maintain the urine pH higher than 6.5 coupled with increased fluid intake. The 24-hour urinary uric acid excretion was normal, so allopurinol was not given. He had no stone recurrence.

PATIENT 3

A 24-year-old man presented with vague flank discomfort. Family history was positive for a sister with kidney stones. Physical examination was remarkable for right costovertebral angle tenderness. A renal ultrasound revealed a moderately radiopaque 2 cm stone in the right kidney. Urinalysis revealed pH of 5 and multiple hexagonal crystals. A 24-hour urine stone risk diagnostic profile was normal. The patient was treated with increased fluid intake, potassium citrate, and nightly acetazolamide. Six months later, the stone had decreased to half its original size.

Q: Why was the urine stone risk profile normal in this patient?

1. There are no metabolic abnormalities
2. The metabolic abnormalities were not detected

A: The hexagonal crystals in this patient are diagnostic of cystinuria. Urine cystine testing is not included in the urine stone risk diagnostic profile as the disorder is rare and the diagnosis can be made on urinalysis.

PATIENT 4

A 40-year-old C5 quadriplegic man with a chronic indwelling urinary catheter presented with urosepsis. His spinal cord injury had been sustained at age 17 during a football practice. After antibiotics were administered, a CT was done, which revealed bilateral staghorn calculi. Urinalysis revealed a urine pH of 9 and coffin-lid crystals. Urine culture grew multiple organisms, including *Proteus*, *Pseudomonas*, *Providencia*, and *Enterococcus* species. He underwent left ESWL (×2) and right ESWL. A 24-hour urine stone risk diagnostic profile was normal.

Q: Which of the following statements is (are) true about struvite stones?

1. Struvite stones only form in the presence of urine infected with a urea-splitting organism
2. Struvite stones frequently present as staghorn calculi
3. Struvite stones can result in end-stage kidney disease
4. All of the above

A: The answer is (4). Struvite, or magnesium ammonium phosphate, can only form in the presence of a urea-splitting organism. Breakdown of urea results in ammonia formation, resulting in alkaline urine that promotes calcium phosphate and/or magnesium ammonium phosphate crystallization. These stones tend to be of the staghorn variety, are difficult to eradicate even with interventional/ surgical procedures, and can cause end-stage kidney disease.

References

Chadwick VS, Modha K, Dowling RH. Mechanism for hyperoxaluria in patients with ileal dysfunction. *N Engl J Med*. 1973;289:172–176.

Coe FL, Lawton RL, Goldstein RB, et al. Sodium urate accelerates precipitation of calcium oxalate in vitro. *Proc Soc Exp Biol Med*. 1975;149:926–929.

Ettinger B, Pak CY, Citron JT, et al. Potassium-magnesium citrate is an effective prophylaxis against recurrent calcium oxalate nephrolithiasis. *J Urol*. 1997;158:2069–2073.

Ettinger B, Tang A, Citron JT, et al. Randomized trial of allopurinol in the prevention of calcium oxalate calculi. *N Engl J Med*. 1986;315:1386–1389.

Laerum E, Larsen S. Thiazide prophylaxis of urolithiasis: a double-blind study in general practice. *Acta Med Scand*. 1984;215:383–389.

Levy FL, Adams-Huet B, Pak CY. Ambulatory evaluation of nephrolithiasis: and update of a 1980 protocol. *Am J Med*. 1995;98(1):50–59.

Marshall RW, Cochran M, Robertson WC, et al. The relation between the concentration of calcium salts in the urine and renal stone composition in patients with calcium-containing renal stones. *Clin Sci*. 1972;43:433–441.

Muldowney FP, Freaney R, Moloney MF. Importance of dietary sodium in the hypercalciuria syndrome. *Kidney Int*. 1982;22:292–296.

Nasr SH, D'Agati VD, Said SM, et al. Oxalate nephropathy complicating Roux-en-Y gastric bypass: an underrecognized cause of irreversible renal failure. *Clin J Am Soc Nephrol*. 2008;3(6): 1676–1683.

Pak CY, Sakhaee K, Crowther C, et al. Evidence justifying a high fluid intake in treatment of nephrolithiasis. *Ann Intern Med*. 1980;93:36–39.

Pak CY, Sakhaee K, Fuller C. Successful management of uric acid nephrolithiasis with potassium citrate. *Kidney Int*. 1986;30:422–428.

Pak CY, Skurla C, Harvey J. Graphic display of urinary risk factors for renal stone formation. *J Urol*. 1985;134:867–870.

Preminger GM. The metabolic evaluation of patients with recurrent nephrolithiasis: a review of comprehensive and simplified approaches. *J Urol*. 1989;141:760–763.

Rodman JS. Struvite stones. *Nephron*. 1999;81(suppl 1):50–59.

Smith LH, Frueth AJ, Hoffman AF. Acquired hyperoxaluria, nephrolithiasis and intestinal disease. *N Engl J Med*. 1972;286:1371–1375.

Yü T, Gutman AB. Uric acid nephrolithiasis in gout. Predisposing factors. *Ann Intern Med*. 1967;67(6):1133–1148.

INDEX

Note: Page numbers followed by *f* indicate figures; those followed by *t* indicate tables.

renal tubular epithelial cell, 7, 9*f,* 10
white blood cells, 6–7, 8*f*
Urinary protein electrophoresis (UPEP), 33
Urine
appearance of, 1–2
dipstick evaluation of, 2–3
microscopic examination of, 4–10, 4–10*f*
Urine albumin-to-creatinine ratio (UACR)
with chronic kidney disease, 32
in clinical medicine, 31–32
vs. urine protein-to-creatinine ratio, 30
Urine anion gap (UAG), 65
use of, 65
utility in diagnosis, 68–71
Urine creatinine, 21
Urine osmolal gap (UOG), 69–70
Urine osmolality (Uosm), 60
Urine protein-to-creatinine ratio (UPCR)
in clinical medicine, 31–32
vs. urine albumin-to-creatinine ratio, 30

Urine-to-plasma creatinine ratio (U/P Cr)
in clinical practice, 37
in healthy people, 35–36
meaning of, 35
Urobilinogen, in urine, 3

V

Vascular calcification
calcium-containing binders, 125, 127
non–calcium-containing binders, 126

W

Water, fractional excretion of, 36
White blood cells
and bacteria., 5*f*
casts, 6–7, 8*f*
in urine, 4, 4*f*

Y

Yeast, in urine, 5